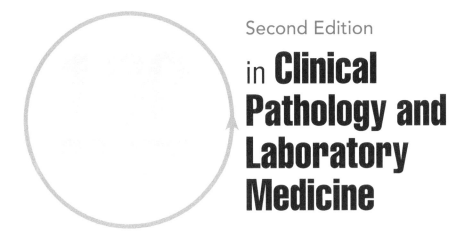

Second Edition

in **Clinical Pathology and Laboratory Medicine**

100 Cases in Clinical Pathology and Laboratory Medicine presents 100 clinical scenarios commonly seen by medical students and junior doctors in the emergency department, outpatient clinic, operating theatre or in general practice. A succinct summary of the patient's history, examination and initial investigations is followed by questions on each case, with particular emphasis on the interpretation of the results and in which an understanding of the underlying clinical pathology is central to arriving at the correct diagnosis. The answer includes a detailed discussion on each topic, providing an essential revision aid, as well as a practical guide for students and junior doctors, especially those preparing for undergraduate and postgraduate examinations.

Making speedy and appropriate clinical decisions, and choosing the best course of action to take as a result, is one of the most important and challenging parts of training to become a doctor. Fully revised and updated for this second edition, these true-to-life cases will teach students and junior doctors to recognise important clinical conditions, to request the appropriate pathological investigations and correctly interpret those results, and, as a result, to develop their diagnostic and management skills.

T0138885

100 Cases
About the Series

Making speedy and appropriate clinical decisions, and choosing the best course of action to take as a result, is one of the most important and challenging parts of training to become a doctor. The real-life cases presented in the 100 Cases series encompass emergency, ward and outpatient and community scenarios, and have been designed specifically to help medical students and junior doctors to develop their diagnostic and management skills.

100 Cases in Clinical Pathology and Laboratory Medicine, 2E
Eamon Shamil, Praful Ravi, Ashish Chandra

100 Cases in Clinical Medicine, 3E
P John Rees, James Pattison, Christopher Kosky

100 Cases in Clinical Pharmacology, Therapeutics and Prescribing
Kerry Layne, Albert Ferro

100 Cases in Dermatology
Rachael Morris-Jones, Ann-Marie Powell, Emma Benton

100 Cases in Emergency Medicine and Critical Care
Eamon Shamil, Praful Ravi, Dipak Mistry

100 Cases in General Practice, 2E
Anne E. Stephenson, Martin Mueller, John Grabinar

100 Cases in Obstetrics and Gynaecology, 2E
Cecilia Bottomley, Janice Rymer

100 Cases in Orthopaedics and Rhematology
Parminder J Singh, Catherine Swales

100 Cases in Paediatrics, 2E
Ronny Cheung, Aubrey Cunnington, Simon Drysdale, Joseph Raine, Joanna Walker

100 Cases in Psychiatry, 2E
Barry Wright, Subodh Dave, Nisha Dogra

100 Cases in Radiology
Robert Thomas, James Connelly, Christopher Burke

100 Cases in Surgery, 2E
James Gossage, Bijan Modarai, Arun Sahai, Richard Worth, Kevin G Burnand

100 Diagnostic Dilemmas in Clinical Medicine
Kerry Layne

For more information about this series please visit: https://www.routledge.com/100-Cases/book-series/CRCONEHUNCAS

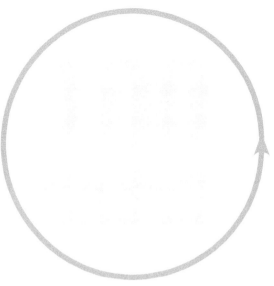

Second Edition

in **Clinical Pathology and Laboratory Medicine**

Eamon Shamil MBBS, MRes, DOHNS, FRCS (ORL-HNS)
Post-CCT Fellow in Rhinology, Anterior Skull Base, and
Facial Plastic Surgery
The Royal National ENT Hospital,
University College London Hospitals NHS
Foundation Trust, UK

Praful Ravi MA, MB, BChir, MRCP
Attending Physician in Genitourinary Oncology,
Dana-Farber Cancer Institute; Instructor of Medicine,
Harvard Medical School, Boston, Massachusetts, USA

Ashish Chandra FRCPath, DipRCPath (Cytol)
Lead Consultant for Cytopathology & Urological
Histopathology, Guy's and St Thomas' NHS Foundation
Trust, London, UK; Chair, British Association of Urological
Pathologists (BAUP); Vice President, International Academy
of Cytology (IAC); Deputy Editor, *Cytopathology*

100 Cases Series Editor:
Janice Rymer MBBS, FRACP
Professor of Obstetrics & Gynaecology and Dean
of Student Affairs, King's College London School
of Medicine, London, UK

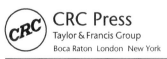

CRC Press
Taylor & Francis Group
Boca Raton London New York

CRC Press is an imprint of the
Taylor & Francis Group, an **informa** business

Second edition published 2023
by CRC Press

6000 Broken Sound Parkway NW, Suite 300, Boca Raton, FL 33487–2742
and by CRC Press

4 Park Square, Milton Park, Abingdon, Oxon, OX14 4RN

CRC Press is an imprint of Taylor & Francis Group, LLC

© 2023 Eamon Shamil, Praful Ravi and Ashish Chandra

First edition published by CRC Press 2014

Library of Congress Cataloging-in-Publication Data
Names: Shamil, Eamon, editor. | Ravi, Praful, editor. | Chandra, Ashish (Histopathologist) editor. |
    Shamil, Eamon. 100 cases in clinical pathology.
Title: 100 cases in clinical pathology and laboratory medicine / edited by Eamon Shamil, Praful Ravi, Ashish Chandra.
    Other titles: One hundred cases in clinical pathology and laboratory medicine | 100 cases
Description: Second edition. | Boca Raton : CRC Press, 2023. | Series: 100 cases | Preceded by 100 cases in clinical
    pathology / Eamon Shamil, Praful Ravi, Ashish Chandra. c2014. | Includes bibliographical references and index. |
    Summary: "100 Cases in Clinical Pathology and Laboratory Medicine presents 100 clinical scenarios commonly
    seen by medical students and junior doctors in the emergency department, outpatient clinic, operating theatre or in
    general practice. A succinct summary of the patient's history, examination and initial investigations is followed by
    questions on each case, with particular emphasis on the interpretation of the results and in which an understanding
    of the underlying clinical pathology is central to arriving at the correct diagnosis. The answer includes a detailed
    discussion on each topic, providing an essential revision aid as well as a practical guide for students and junior
    doctors, especially those preparing for undergraduate and postgraduate examinations. Making speedy and
    appropriate clinical decisions, and choosing the best course of action to take as a result, is one of the most important
    and challenging parts of training to become a doctor. Fully revised and updated for this second edition, these
    true-to-life cases will teach students and junior doctors to recognize important clinical conditions, to request the
    appropriate pathological investigation and correctly interpret those results, and, as a result, to develop their
    diagnostic and management skills"— Provided by publisher.
Identifiers: LCCN 2022032063 (print) | LCCN 2022032064 (ebook) | ISBN 9781032151397 (hardback) |
    ISBN 9781032151373 (paperback) | ISBN 9781003242697 (ebook)
Subjects: MESH: Pathologic Processes | Signs and Symptoms | Clinical Laboratory Techniques | Problems and
    Exercises | Case Reports
Classification: LCC RC69 (print) | LCC RC69 (ebook) | NLM QZ 18.2 | DDC 616/.047—dc23/eng/20220914
LC record available at https://lccn.loc.gov/2022032063
LC ebook record available at https://lccn.loc.gov/2022032064

ISBN: 9781032151397 (hbk)
ISBN: 9781032151373 (pbk)
ISBN: 9781003242697 (ebk)

DOI: 10.1201/9781003242697

Typeset in Baskerville
by Apex CoVantage, LLC

Access the Support Material: www.routledge.com/9781032151373

CONTENTS

Section 1: Laboratory Medicine: Chemical Pathology, Immunology and Genetics

Section 2: Histopathology

Section 3: Haematology

Section 4: Microbiology

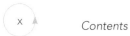

Bonus cases are available for download at: www.routledge.com/9781032151373

PREFACE

We are pleased to present a second edition of this textbook, having received excellent feedback on the first edition, which was published in 2014. We have revised the cases and included new ones to reflect the updated medical student curriculum. We have also updated the name of the textbook to include Laboratory Medicine, reflecting content that explains how to interpret and manage abnormal blood tests.

Our aim remains the same: to improve the understanding of the underlying pathology of both common and rare (but important) conditions. We explain how the underlying pathology is related to symptoms, investigations, and management of patients, giving the reader a useful overview of the topic, as well as preparing them for undergraduate and postgraduate exams. An appreciation for "how does this disease process occur" will help students and doctors provide better care to their patients and drive enthusiasm to improve care.

Eamon Shamil
Praful Ravi
Ashish Chandra

ACKNOWLEDGEMENTS

The specimen images are from the Gordon Museum of Pathology, King's College London.

CONTRIBUTORS

Dr Mark Ong BSc, MBChB, MRCS
Consultant Histopathologist
Guy's & St Thomas' NHS Foundation Trust
London, UK

Dr Alexander Polson FRCPath
Consultant Histopathologist
Guy's & St Thomas' NHS Foundation Trust
London, UK

Dr Caryn Rosmarin MBBCh, DTM&H, MSc (Med Micro), FCPath (SA), FRCPath
Microbiology/Infection Control Consultant
Microbiology Training Programme Director (NE London)
Barts Health NHS Trust
London, UK

Dr Simran Goyal BA, MBBCh
Foundation Doctor
School of Clinical Medicine
University of Cambridge, UK

Dr Hassen al-Sader MBBS, MRCP
Haematology Consultant
West Hertfordshire Teaching Hospitals NHS Trust
Honorary Consultant, Lymphoma Team, University College London Hospital, UK

Dr Wael Faroug Elamin MBBS, BSc, MSc, MD, FRCPath, FRCP.
Medical Director, G42 Healthcare,UAE;
Honorary Senior Lecturer, QMUL;
Consultant Clinical Microbiologist, Elrazi University, Sudan

REFERENCE RANGES

HAEMATOLOGY

Haemoglobin (Hb)	11.4–15.0 g/dL
White cells (WCC)	3.9–10.6 g/dL
Neutrophils	$2.0–7.5 \times 10_9$/L
Lymphocytes	$1.3–3.5 \times 10_9$/L
Eosinophils	$<0.4 \times 10_9$/L
Platelets (PLT)	$150–440 \times 10_9$/L
Reticulocytes	0.5–1.5%
Mean cell volume (MCV)	77–95 fL
Mean cell haemoglobin (MCH)	27.0–32.0 pg
Serum iron	14–31 mmol/L
Serum ferritin	20–300 mg/L
Total iron binding capacity (TIBC)	45–80 µmol/L
Transferrin saturation	20–50%

BIOCHEMISTRY

Sodium (Na)	135–145 mmol/L
Potassium (K)	3.5–5 mmol/L
Urea (Ur)	2.5–7.8 mmol/L
Creatinine (Cr)	60–110 µmol/L
Fasting glucose (Gluc)	3.5–6 mmol/L
Bilirubin (Bili)	<21 µmol/L
Alanine aminotransferase (ALT)	10–40 IU/L
Aspartate aminotransferase (AST)	11–60 IU/L
Alkaline phosphatase (ALP)	20–140 IU/L
Gamma glutamyl transferase (GGT)	<65 IU/L
Serum protein	60–80 g/L
Albumin (Alb)	35–50 g/L
Corrected calcium (corr Ca)	2.1–2.6 mmol/L
Phosphate (PO_4)	0.81–1.45 mmol/L
Parathyroid hormone (PTH)	1.2–5.8 pmol/L
Prolactin (non-pregnant)	<20 ng/mL
Serum osmolality	278–305 mOsm/kg
Lactate dehydrogenase (LDH)	240–480 IU/L
IgG	6.5–16.0 g/L
IgA	0.4–3.5 g/L
IgM	0.55–3.0 g/L
C-reactive protein (CRP)	<5 mg/L
Erythrocyte sedimentation rate (ESR)	<30 mm/hr
Thyroid-stimulating hormone (TSH)	0.5–5 mU/L
Total T4	58–174 nmol/L
Free T4	10–23 pmol/L
Free T3	3.5–6.5 pmol/L

Amylase   60–180 U/L
Cholesterol   <5 mmol/L
LDL cholesterol   <3 mmol/L
HDL cholesterol   >1 mmol/L
Triglyceride   <2.26 mmol/L

COAGULATION

International normalised ratio (INR)   0.9–1.2 sec
Prothrombin time (PT)   11–15 sec
Activated partial thromboplastin time (APTT)   18–28 sec
Fibrinogen   1.5–3.0 g/L
D-Dimer   <250 µg/L

URINE

Urine osmolality   50–1200 mOsm/kg
Urine pH   6.5–8

BLOOD GASES

pH   7.35–7.45
pO_2 11.3–12.6 kPa
pCO_2 4.5–6 kPa
HCO_3 –22 to 26 mmol/L
Base excess   –2 to 2 mmol/L

Section 1
LABORATORY MEDICINE: CHEMICAL PATHOLOGY, IMMUNOLOGY AND GENETICS

CASE 1: POLYURIA AND POLYDIPSIA

A 45-year-old woman with a history of hypothyroidism presents to her GP with a 3-month history of urinary frequency, up to three times per night. She finds that her constant desire to drink fluids, particularly cold water, and her frequent need to visit the toilet interfere with her job as a teacher. She has no other health problems and has no regular medications.

Examination

The patient looks well, with no evidence of dehydration. Examination of her heart, lungs and abdomen is unremarkable. Neurologic examination is normal. Urine dipstick is negative.

🔍 INVESTIGATIONS

Haemoglobin	13.5
White cells	8.3
Platelets	325
Sodium	144
Potassium	4.2
Urea	6.5
Creatinine	100
Fasting glucose	6.0
Corrected calcium	2.25

A water deprivation test is performed, as shown in Figure 1.1.

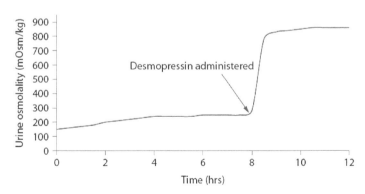

Figure 1.1 A water deprivation test.

? **QUESTIONS**

1. What is the differential diagnosis, and what further tests are required?
2. What is the principle of a water deprivation test, and how do you interpret her results?
3. Discuss the pathophysiology of the likely diagnosis and suggest how the patient may be treated.

ANSWERS

This woman presents with polyuria, nocturia and polydipsia. These symptoms have four important differential diagnoses: (1) diabetes mellitus; (2) diabetes insipidus, which may either be central or nephrogenic in origin; (3) hypercalcaemia, which may present like the above in an acute setting; and (4) primary polydipsia (PP). Therefore, investigations need to be directed at elucidating one of the above diagnoses.

Diabetes insipidus is a relatively rare disease characterised by the excretion of large volumes of dilute urine as a result of either a deficiency of or a resistance to the actions of the posterior pituitary hormone, antidiuretic hormone (ADH), also known as arginine vasopressin (AVP). ADH is released into the circulation from the posterior pituitary gland in response to an increase in serum osmolality and acts to increase reabsorption of water by inserting aquaporin-2 (AQP2) channels into the apical membrane of the distal parts of the nephron. Deficiency of ADH leads to central diabetes insipidus (CDI), while failure of the kidney to respond to its actions causes nephrogenic diabetes insipidus (NDI).

Diagnosis of diabetes insipidus includes basic laboratory investigations and a fluid deprivation test. Hypernatraemia may be found secondary to dehydration, while urinalysis may show a low specific gravity (<1.005). Serum osmolality is increased due to excess free water loss. It may be formally measured or estimated using the formula: $2 \times [Na^+] + [urea] + [glucose]$, which would be around 300 mOsm/kg in this patient. Similarly, urine osmolality will be low, generally less than 200 mOsm/kg, due to inadequate reabsorption of water from the distal parts of the nephron.

When the diagnosis is equivocal, a fluid deprivation test may be performed. Patients are deprived of fluid intake for a period of 8 hours, with hourly measurement of body weight, urine volume and urine osmolality. After allowing a sufficient time for dehydration, desmopressin (synthetic ADH) is administered subcutaneously, and a final urine sample is taken 1 hour afterwards to measure urine osmolality.

The essence of the test is that with CDI, urine will become more concentrated once the deficient ADH is replaced, whereas with NDI, the inability of the kidney to respond to ADH means that any further replacement by ADH has no effect.

CDI is commonly idiopathic. However, autoantibodies against ADH-secreting cells of the hypothalamus may be detected, especially if the patient exhibits other autoimmune conditions, such as hypothyroidism, as in this case. Other causes of CDI include brain tumours, such as germinomas and craniopharyngiomas; neurosurgery; head injury; and infiltrative conditions, such as Langerhans cell histiocytosis. There are also genetic forms of the disease, with the majority being inherited in an autosomal dominant fashion with mutations in the ADH gene.

CDI responds well to ADH replacement, usually via the synthetic analogue desmopressin (DDAVP). High-dose DDAVP may be used for mild cases of NDI, but treatment of NDI requires management of the underlying cause (e.g., correcting metabolic abnormalities, discontinuing any offending drugs). In any case, treatment is required only if the patient is suffering from severe dehydration, with urine volumes >4 L per day.

🔑 KEY POINTS

- Causes of polyuria and polydipsia include diabetes mellitus, diabetes insipidus, hypercalcaemia and PP.
- Diabetes insipidus is due either to inadequate central production of ADH or failure of the kidneys to respond to ADH.
- Central diabetes insipidus is frequently idiopathic and managed with synthetic ADH (desmopressin).

CASE 2: TRACES OF BLOOD FOUND ON URINE DIPSTICK

A 60-year-old office executive presents to his GP for his yearly 'well man' check. He reports no significant health problems. He has a history of hypertension treated with lisinopril, type 2 diabetes controlled by diet and exercise and benign prostatic hyperplasia (BPH), for which he takes tamsulosin. He has a family history of prostate cancer, in his father and two paternal uncles. He has a 20 pack-year smoking history.

Examination

Physical examination is unremarkable. Digital rectal examination confirms a large, smooth prostate. Urine dipstick shows ++ blood, but no other abnormalities.

? QUESTIONS

1. What are the causes of non-visible haematuria?
2. What features in the history might warrant the haematuria to be further investigated by the GP or merit referral to secondary care?
3. What investigations need to be performed in the Urology clinic to elucidate the cause in this patient?

ANSWERS

Haematuria is classified as either visible or non-visible, with the latter defined as the presence of 3–5 red blood cells per high power field on urine microscopy on at least two of three examinations over a period of 2–3 weeks. Visible haematuria is less prevalent than non-visible haematuria and is defined as a single observation of gross urine discolouration by blood. While the same pathologies may cause either visible or non-visible haematuria, the relative frequency of these causes varies between the two.

The causes of non-visible haematuria are:

1. Glomerular (e.g., glomerulonephritis, immunoglobulin A [IgA] nephropathy, hereditary causes)
2. Non-glomerular
   a. Upper urinary tract (nephrolithiasis, pyelonephritis, renal cell carcinoma, cystic disease of the kidney, renal trauma, metabolic derangements such as hypercalciuria)
   b. Lower urinary tract (bladder and prostate cancer, benign lesions such as BPH and bladder papillomas, urethritis, cystitis)
3. Other (e.g., excess anticoagulation, 'march' haematuria)

Malignancy and urolithiasis are the underlying cause in 10% of patients, while a significant proportion of cases turn out to be unexplainable. Glomerular and non-glomerular causes may be distinguished by the presence of proteinuria, which is often found in the former but not the latter.

While an isolated dipstick-positive haematuria does not necessarily merit immediate further evaluation, features in the history may help the GP decide whether to investigate further— the family history of prostate cancer, as well as the patient's history of BPH and smoking history, would be worrying features. The GP should also look for causes such as exercise, recent sexual activity, or any trauma to the urinary tract.

Evaluation of haematuria in secondary care occurs in a systematic manner, with 'one-stop' haematuria clinics becoming the norm. Urine dipstick, microscopy and culture are required, and renal function should be assessed. In the presence of proteinuria and deranged renal function, referral to a nephrologist is merited since a glomerular cause is likely. Urine microscopy helps to confirm haematuria, as well as looking for potential clues to the cause (e.g., red cell casts in glomerulonephritis), while culture will identify infection.

Workup then proceeds to the upper and lower urinary tracts. The cornerstone of upper urinary tract investigation is imaging via ultrasound or CT urogram; CT is preferred, as it has higher sensitivity and specificity. In around 30% of patients, these investigations will identify a cause; the remainder require lower urinary tract investigations. Urine cytology is required to look for urothelial malignancy, and cystoscopy should be considered, as it has higher sensitivity than cytology for diagnosing bladder cancer. It is generally recommended for all patients with non-visible haematuria over the age of 40 and for anyone with risk factors for bladder malignancy.

🔑 KEY POINTS

- Haematuria has a number of causes and should always be taken seriously.
- Investigation of haematuria includes urinary testing, assessment of renal function, imaging of the upper urinary tract and possibly cystoscopy.
- Painless haematuria should raise the suspicion of bladder cancer.

CASE 3: CONFUSION, LETHARGY AND SHORTNESS OF BREATH

A retired 68-year-old man is admitted to the medical assessment unit with a 3-month history of progressive shortness of breath, lethargy and recent-onset confusion. He is now short of breath at rest and has noted that he has very little energy. His past medical history includes chronic obstructive pulmonary disease and mild hypertension. He has a 20 pack-year smoking history.

Examination

His respiratory rate is 24, O_2 saturation of 94% on room air. Breath sounds are reduced in the right mid-zone. His jugular venous pulse (JVP) is not elevated, and there is no peripheral oedema.

🔍 INVESTIGATIONS

Haemoglobin	12.2
White cells	8.5
Platelets	350
Sodium	127
Potassium	4.5
Urea	5
Creatinine	100
C-reactive protein	20
Serum osmolality	260 mOsm
Urine osmolality	250 mOsm
Urine Na	50 mM
Chest radiograph: Ill-defined opacity in the right perihilar region	

? QUESTIONS

1. What are the possible causes of hyponatraemia?
2. What is the likely diagnosis and underlying pathophysiology in this case?
3. How should the patient be managed next?

ANSWERS

Hyponatraemia is defined as a serum sodium concentration of less than 135 mM. It is a common problem, particularly in hospitalised patients, and is generally a secondary phenomenon to an underlying pathologic or physiologic process.

Plasma osmolality may be increased, normal, or decreased in hyponatraemia, and is reduced in the majority of cases. Hypertonic hyponatraemia arises when solutes in the extracellular fluid (as occurring with hyperglycaemia or with hypertonic mannitol infusion) draw water across from cells. Isotonic hyponatraemia usually arises with retention of isosmotic fluid in the extracellular space (e.g., isotonic glucose infusion) or when severe hyperlipidaemia or hyperproteinaemia reduces the fractional water content, leading to a 'pseudohyponatraemia'. Hypotonic hyponatraemia is most common. This may be in the presence of a reduced, normal or increased extracellular fluid volume. Hypovolaemic hyponatraemia is caused by sodium depletion, either by renal or extra-renal means. Hypervolaemic hyponatraemia occurs with retention of sodium and water, which is due to activation of the renin-angiotensin-aldosterone axis secondary to heart failure, cirrhosis or nephrotic syndrome.

This patient's fluid status appears normal, indicating the presence of euvolaemic hyponatraemia. Here, sodium content is diluted by water excess, the causes of which include syndrome of inappropriate antidiuretic hormone (SIADH), hypothyroidism and a reduced intake of solutes.

SIADH is the most frequent cause of hyponatraemia and describes a condition where antidiuretic hormone (ADH) levels are inappropriately high for the plasma osmolality. The key diagnostic criteria for SIADH are (1) reduced plasma osmolality <275 mOsm, (2) urine osmolality >100 mOsm, (3) clinical euvolaemia and (4) continued natriuresis >40 mM in the presence of (5) normal thyroid and adrenal function and (6) without recent use of diuretics. Common conditions causing SIADH include malignancy (especially small cell lung cancer), lung disease (including pneumonia, tuberculosis [TB] and cystic fibrosis), cranial disease (encephalitis, meningitis and trauma), and drugs (e.g., selective serotonin reuptake inhibitors [SSRIs] and antipsychotics).

Here, the history of lethargy and shortness of breath in a smoker together with a suspicious chest radiograph suggests a paraneoplastic process. Small cell lung cancers are thought to arise from neuroendocrine progenitor cells of the lining of the bronchial epithelium and can secrete high levels of ADH with resultant hyponatraemia.

The management of SIADH is directed at the underlying cause—in this case, this would involve management (typically via chemotherapy) of the lung malignancy. In the short term, fluid restriction is the cornerstone of treatment; the aim should be to gradually correct the electrolyte abnormality since too rapid a correction can lead to osmotic demyelination in the central nervous system (central pontine myelinolysis).

🔑 KEY POINTS

- When faced with hyponatraemia, first ask yourself whether plasma osmolality is reduced, increased or normal.
- The most common cause of hypotonic hyponatraemia where fluid status is normal is SIADH.
- In addition to treating the underlying cause, patients with SIADH require fluid restriction.

CASE 4: A CHILD WITH FACIAL SWELLING

A 7-year-old boy is brought into the emergency department by his mother, as she has noticed his face swelling up in the past week. Apart from a sore throat 2 weeks ago, the boy has been fit and well, though he has felt a bit 'off colour' since the minor illness and has reported that his urine has become bubbly.

Examination
Physical examination reveals a well-looking child with bilateral periorbital oedema and bilateral pitting pedal oedema.

INVESTIGATIONS

Sodium	135
Potassium	3.8
Urea	3
Creatinine	85
Albumin	24
Corrected calcium	2.05
Urine dipstick: +++ protein, no blood	

QUESTIONS

1. What is the term given to the spectrum of findings described above, and what further investigations should be performed?
2. What are the possible causes in this particular case, and which is most likely?
3. What is the pathophysiology of the most likely cause, and what should the mother be told about the likely prognosis?

ANSWERS

The spectrum of findings found in this patient, namely proteinuria, hypoalbuminaemia and oedema, is called nephrotic syndrome. The initiating event is the leakage of large amounts of protein (>3.5 g per day) in urine, which results in hypoalbuminaemia. The subsequent fall in plasma oncotic pressure leads to redistribution of extracellular fluid to the interstitial compartment, producing oedema. *Nephrotic* syndrome should be distinguished from *nephritic* syndrome, the latter representing an inflammatory process often characterised by haematuria, uraemia and a degree of renal failure, whereas the former typically represents a degenerative process.

There are numerous consequences of proteinuria, which need to be the subject of further investigations. The hypoalbuminaemic state provokes an increased rate of hepatic protein synthesis, which leads to hyperlipidaemia and, on occasion, lipiduria. The loss of protein leads to other metabolic derangements as well, principally hypocalcaemia. Nephrotic syndrome is also associated with a hypercoagulable state, with a particular association with renal vein thrombosis. The cause for this is unclear, but hypotheses include (1) excess loss of anticoagulant factors (such as protein S and antithrombin) in urine and increased production of procoagulant factors (such as factors V and VIII) by the liver; (2) increased platelet aggregation; (3) immune complex–mediated injury to the glomerulus, causing a procoagulant effect; and (4) increased production of lipoprotein (a).

The causes of nephrotic syndrome may be grouped into two categories:

1. Primary glomerular disorders, such as minimal change disease (MCD), membranous glomerulopathy, focal segmental glomerulosclerosis (FSGS) and other glomerulonephritides
2. Systemic diseases affecting the kidney, such as diabetes mellitus, amyloidosis, systemic lupus erythematosus and medications (e.g., non-steroidal anti-inflammatory drugs [NSAIDs]).

The most common cause of nephrotic syndrome in children is MCD. Here, the history of an upper respiratory tract infection is suggestive of MCD given the temporal association between the two.

The term *minimal change disease* refers to the fact that the histologic appearance of nephrons in diseased individuals looks normal. However, on electron microscopy, effacement of podocyte foot processes in the glomerulus is observed. The pathogenesis of MCD is uncertain, with the most popular theory proposing that it arises as a disorder of T-cell function, with release of several cytokines, such as interleukin (IL)-4, IL-10 and IL-13, that injure the glomerulus.

Treatment of the first attack of MCD is via steroids, typically for a period of around 6–8 weeks, and the majority of children achieve a complete remission. Relapses may be treated with steroids, or, in refractory cases, with immunosuppressants such as cyclophosphamide or cyclosporine. In any case, the majority of children with MCD stop having relapses and live a normal life without any evidence of renal failure or urinary abnormalities.

> 🔑 **KEY POINTS**
>
> - Nephrotic syndrome is characterised by proteinuria, hypoalbuminaemia and oedema.
> - The most common cause of nephrotic syndrome in a child is MCD.
> - Treatment of MCD principally involves use of corticosteroids, and most children can be anticipated to make a full recovery with retention of normal renal function.

CASE 5: JOINT PAINS AND FATIGUE

A 35-year-old woman of Indian origin is referred to a rheumatology clinic with a 6-month history of persistent joint pain in her right fingers and left wrist and intermittent headaches not responsive to analgesia. She also reports a generalised feeling of fatigue. She has no relevant past medical history. Family history is notable for hypothyroidism in her mother. She takes folic acid, as she is trying to conceive, having suffered a recent miscarriage.

Examination

Musculoskeletal examination is positive for tenderness in her right metacarpophalangeal joints as well as the left radiocarpal joint. Neurologic examination is unremarkable. Urine dipstick shows trace of protein and blood.

INVESTIGATIONS

Haemoglobin	10.8
White cells	9.8
Platelets	160
Mean cell volume	95
Sodium	140
Potassium	4.2
Urea	5.6
Creatinine	90
Bilirubin	10
Alanine aminotransferase	40
Aspartate aminotransferase	35
Alkaline phosphatase	85
Lactate dehydrogenase	340
Thyroid-stimulating hormone	3.8
International normalised ratio	1.1
Glucose (random)	6.8
Antinuclear antibody	Positive

QUESTIONS

1. What is your differential diagnosis?
2. What further investigations would you request?
3. What are the common complications of this condition?

ANSWERS

The key features in this history are arthralgia, headache and fatigue, which are non-specific and give a wide differential. However, the examination findings and investigations reduce the number of possibilities significantly. The investigations reveal a normocytic anaemia with an elevated lactate dehydrogenase (LDH), possibly suggesting haemolytic anaemia, with a borderline thrombocytopenia and positive antinuclear antibody (ANA) test, against the background of normal thyroid, renal and liver function. ANA positivity is not specific for any particular autoimmune disease but does raise this possibility. In this case, ANA positivity points towards a differential of autoimmune or connective tissue disorders, including systemic lupus erythematosus (SLE), scleroderma, rheumatoid arthritis, mixed connective tissue disease, Sjögren's syndrome and inflammatory myopathies such as dermatomyositis and polymyositis.

This patient meets the 2019 European Alliance of Associations for Rheumatology/American College of Rheumatology (EULAR/ACR) classification criteria for the diagnosis of SLE, as she has a positive ANA along with (1) arthritis, (2) neurologic symptoms and (3) haemolytic anaemia. While SLE can be putatively diagnosed with these conditions, further investigations would be useful in confirming this. In particular, specific autoantibodies for SLE (e.g., anti-dsDNA and anti-SmAg) would be helpful in making the diagnosis. Given the history of a miscarriage, antiphospholipid antibodies could be tested to exclude lupus anticoagulant syndrome.

The pathogenesis of SLE is not well understood, with genetic, environmental, hormonal and immunoregulatory factors all playing a part in the ultimate breakdown of self-tolerance, which leads to organ injury. One theory is that a defect in clearance of apoptotic or necrotic cells leads to the sensitisation of T and B cells to intracellular antigens, triggering the autoimmune process. For example, deficiencies of early complement components (C1q, C4), which are important for these clearance processes, produce an SLE-like syndrome. Other hypotheses include aberrant T-cell signal transduction, as well as overexpression of particular cytokines (in particular, type I interferons).

Tissue injury in SLE is immune complex mediated (type III hypersensitivity) as a result of defective clearance of apoptotic or necrotic cells due to deficiency of Fc and complement receptors. The most important complication arises in the kidney, where immune complex accumulation stimulates secretion of pro-inflammatory cytokines by mesangial cells and podocytes, giving rise to lupus nephritis. About 50% of patients develop clinically evident renal disease, which carries substantial morbidity if severe. Further complications of SLE include an increased cardiovascular risk due to accelerated atherogenesis arising from inflammatory damage to the endothelium. While the prognosis is variable, depending on the extent of organ involvement, current treatments are reasonably effective, with 10-year overall survival greater than 90%.

🔑 **KEY POINTS**

- A positive ANA does not definitively indicate the presence of an autoimmune condition but should prompt suspicion of such.
- SLE is a multi-system autoimmune disorder whose presentation is protean.
- The most important complication of SLE is kidney damage, which may affect up to half of all patients and carries substantial morbidity.

CASE 6: ANXIETY, IRRITABILITY AND REDUCED MENSTRUAL FREQUENCY

An otherwise healthy 32-year-old woman presents to the general medical clinic with a feeling of being 'on edge' for 3 months. She also reports difficulty sleeping, increased irritability, 'grittiness' in her eyes and reduced frequency of her periods. She has lost 5 kg in weight over the same period. Family history is notable for rheumatoid arthritis in her mother.

Examination

Her pulse is 90 and regular, and she has warm, slightly sweaty peripheries along with a fine bilateral tremor. Proptosis is noted, and a diffusely enlarged thyroid is palpable.

 INVESTIGATIONS

Serum thyroid-stimulating hormone <0.01, free T4 35, free T3 16

? QUESTIONS

1. Suggest a differential diagnosis in this patient. Which is most likely?
2. Discuss the pathophysiology of the likely diagnosis, and suggest further investigations that may be useful.
3. What is the explanation for the visual signs and symptoms?
4. Outline a preliminary management plan for this patient.

DOI: 10.1201/9781003242697-7

ANSWERS

The cardiovascular, neurologic, reproductive and metabolic findings are classic symptoms of a thyrotoxic state. Hyperthyroidism specifically refers to the increased production of thyroid hormone by the thyroid gland, and the suppressed thyroid-stimulating hormone (TSH) level and high levels of T4 and T3 confirm that it is the cause of thyrotoxicosis here. The most important causes of hyperthyroidism are:

- Autoimmune disease (Graves' disease)
- Thyroidal autonomy (e.g., toxic multinodular goitre, toxic adenoma, functional thyroid carcinoma)
- Inflammatory conditions affecting the thyroid (e.g., painless thyroiditis, subacute thyroiditis)
- Exogenous source of thyroid hormone (e.g., 'hamburger' thyrotoxicosis, surreptitious use of thyroxine)
- Drug-induced (e.g., amiodarone, radiographic contrast dyes)

The features of hyperthyroidism, the presence of eye disease, a diffusely enlarged thyroid and the absence of any history of drug use or recent infection are all suggestive of Graves' disease, which is the underlying cause of 50–80% of cases of hyperthyroidism.

Graves' disease affects less than 1% of the population, with a 5:1 female preponderance. It is an autoimmune disorder where autoantibodies against various proteins (including the TSH receptor, thyroid peroxidase enzyme and thyroglobulin) bind and activate the TSH receptor. This stimulates thyroid follicular hyperplasia and hypertrophy, leading to diffuse thyroid enlargement and increased thyroid hormone synthesis.

Further investigations that may help support the diagnosis of Graves' disease include measurement of autoantibodies, though these are not formally needed for diagnosis.

Testing for ophthalmopathy is important in Graves' disease, as the eyes are affected in 50% of cases, and the condition is serious enough to threaten sight loss in 2–3%. The pathophysiology is uncertain but is thought to be due to autoreactive T cells reacting against antigens in the eye, causing the activation of orbital fibroblasts with subsequent synthesis of extracellular matrix. These serve to displace the eyeball forward and may interfere with the function of the extraocular muscles.

The management options for Graves' hyperthyroidism include anti-thyroid drugs, radioiodine treatment and surgery. Randomised data have shown that all three are equally effective, with anti-thyroid drugs (e.g., carbimazole) preferred as initial management in Europe. Beta-blockers may be used to provide rapid symptomatic relief prior to initiation of definitive management.

 KEY POINTS

- Hyperthyroidism specifically refers to increased production of thyroid hormone by the thyroid gland and is the most common cause of thyrotoxicosis.
- Graves' disease is the most frequent cause of hyperthyroidism and is an autoimmune disorder where autoantibodies stimulate the TSH receptor.
- Ophthalmopathy is an important complication of Graves' disease and may be due to T cells reacting against retro-orbital antigens.

CASE 7: SCREENING FOR PROSTATE CANCER

A 55-year-old Caucasian man presents to his GP with questions on a recent news article that he has read on prostate cancer screening. As he has a family history of the disease (his father and uncle were both diagnosed with the disease in their 70s), he wishes to undergo screening for the disease via prostate specific antigen (PSA) measurement. He does not complain of any lower urinary tract symptoms. He has a background of diet-controlled diabetes mellitus and hypertension, for which he takes amlodipine.

Examination

Cardiac, respiratory and abdominal examinations are unremarkable. On digital rectal examination, the GP finds what he believes to be a benign-feeling prostate.

 INVESTIGATIONS

The patient's most recent full blood count and renal function are within normal limits.

? QUESTIONS

1. Describe the principles of screening and what criteria are used to determine the quality of a screening test.
2. What is the PSA screening test, and what are the ways in which it may be used in a more accurate fashion?
3. What is the current evidence on PSA screening for prostate cancer? Would you recommend it in this case?

DOI: 10.1201/9781003242697-8

ANSWERS

Screening is a public health service where members of the whole population are offered a test that helps identify those at higher risk of the disease so that they may undergo further testing. In the UK, screening takes place from birth to older age, including programmes such as fetal anomaly testing, infectious diseases in pregnancy, the newborn blood spot, diabetic eye screening and cancer screening (bowel, breast and cervical). The criteria for a suitable screening test, as defined by Wilson and Jungner for the World Health Organization in 1968, state that:

- The disease being screened should be an important health problem.
- The natural history of the disease should be well understood.
- There should be an identifiable early stage of disease.
- Treatment at an early stage should be of more benefit than at a later stage.
- There should be a suitable test to identify the early stage.
- The test should be acceptable to the population.
- The intervals for repeating the test should be well defined.
- Suitable facilities should exist to account for the workload resulting from screening.
- Risks of the test, both physical and psychological, should be less than the anticipated benefits.
- Costs should be balanced against benefits.

Prostate cancer is the most common male cancer and the second leading cause of cancer death in men in the UK. PSA is an enzyme produced by the prostate gland whose purpose is to liquefy semen, and normally, only very small levels of PSA are found in serum. Elevated levels may be found in men with prostate cancer, along with other benign conditions, such as benign prostatic hyperplasia (BPH), prostatitis, and after digital rectal examination and ejaculation. As a crude measure, PSA may therefore not be very accurate as a screening measure for prostate cancer. However, it may be used in a better fashion through calculation of PSA density (which corrects for prostate volume), PSA velocity (the rate of the rise in PSA is greater in malignancy), age-specific PSA ranges, and the ratio between free and bound PSA in serum (in general, the percentage of free PSA is lower in cancer). Despite these modifications, PSA screening for prostate cancer is not currently recommended by the National Institute for Health and Clinical Excellence (NICE) in the UK.

The current evidence on PSA screening is very controversial. A large European randomised study found that although PSA screening did significantly reduce mortality from prostate cancer, more than 1000 men would have to be screened and 37 cancers would need to be detected in order to prevent one death from prostate cancer over 11 years of follow-up. In contrast, an American randomised trial found that PSA screening did not achieve a reduction in mortality from prostate cancer, though this study was hampered by the fact that a significant proportion of men in the control (the non-PSA screened arm) did actually undergo a PSA test at some point during the study period. There is also growing data to support use of MRI to complement PSA testing as a means of screening men for prostate cancer.

🔑 **KEY POINTS**

- The purpose of screening is to identify individuals at increased risk of disease so that they may undergo further testing.
- Criteria for a screening test include the condition being an important health problem and there being an identifiable early stage of disease.

CASE 8: A YOUNG WOMAN IS FOUND UNCONSCIOUS IN BED

A 27-year-old woman is brought into the emergency department by her husband, who found her unconscious in bed. The paramedics perform an ABCDE assessment and find her finger-prick glucose to be 1.2 mM. Administration of 50 mL of 20% dextrose revives her. In hospital, the patient gives a history of awakening that morning with a headache but not being able to remember anything else. She has no past medical history, and family history is positive for 'thyroid problems' in her mother. She is a non-smoker and drinks alcohol only socially, though she does confess to drinking large amounts of Coca-Cola every day.

Examination
Cardiac, respiratory, abdominal and neurologic examinations are all unremarkable.

INVESTIGATIONS

FBC, U+E	Normal
Random glucose	5.5 mM
Thyroid-stimulating hormone	2 mU/L
Short Synacthen test	Within normal limits

Given the history of a hypoglycaemic episode, a supervised fast is performed. At the start of the fast (8 am), plasma glucose is 5.4 mM, falling to 4.2 mM at noon, and then 2.3 mM at 4 pm, before reaching a nadir of 1.8 mM at 6 pm. At that time the fast is stopped, and levels of insulin and C-peptide taken at this point are 70 pM (5–20) and 25 nM (0.2–0.9), respectively.

QUESTIONS

1. What are the causes of the patient's hypoglycaemic state?
2. Explain the rationale for the investigations performed in this case. Why would the physician feel confident of a diagnosis at the end of these?
3. What further tests are required at this stage with regard to forming a management plan for the patient?
4. What are the principles of treatment in this case, and how should the patient be treated while awaiting her definitive management?
5. What follow-up should the patient receive?

ANSWERS

Blood glucose level is determined by the balance between insulin and the counter-regulatory hormones (glucagon, adrenaline, growth hormone and cortisol), with hypoglycaemia arising when the balance is shifted too far towards the latter. The clinical features of hypoglycaemia are divided into either autonomic or neurologic symptoms. This presentation highlights the neuroglycopaenic symptoms (e.g., blurred vision, amnesia, loss of consciousness) that occur as a result of a deficient supply of glucose to the brain. The responses of glucagon and adrenaline to a low-glucose state are responsible for the symptoms of autonomic hyper-reactivity, such as sweating, tremor, nausea and palpitations.

Symptomatic hypoglycaemia has several causes, which may be broadly classified as either fasting or non-fasting. Non-fasting hypoglycaemia occurs after a meal; possible causes of this include (1) gastrectomy or alimentary bypass surgery resulting in rapid gastric emptying, leading to overproduction of insulin; (2) pancreatic islet cell hyperplasia; and (3) occult diabetes, which may produce late hypoglycaemia after a meal owing to the deficient early response of insulin in diabetics, leading to exaggerated delayed release 4–5 hours afterwards.

The causes of fasting hypoglycaemia include:

1. Hyperinsulinaemic states
   a. Insulin reaction or sulphonylurea overdose (the most common cause)
   b. Autoimmune hypoglycaemia
   c. Surreptitious use of insulin or sulphonylureas
   d. Pancreatic β-cell tumours (typically insulinoma)
2. Non-hyperinsulinaemic states
   a. Reduced hepatic gluconeogenesis, which may arise from liver disease or inborn errors of metabolism
   b. Renal insufficiency (the kidney contributes to gluconeogenesis too)
   c. Alcohol excess, which increases the activity of alcohol dehydrogenase (consuming NAD^+) and thereby limits the conversion of lactate to pyruvate, which is a gluconeogenic substrate
   d. Non-pancreatic tumours (e.g., retroperitoneal fibrosarcoma) that release insulin-like growth factor (IGF)-2, which can activate the insulin receptor

This patient has fasting hypoglycaemia (a clue is the persistent drinking of Coca-Cola as a subconscious defence against this), and the absence of other causes point towards a hyper-insulinaemic state as the cause. If we assume that the patient has not been using insulin or other antidiabetic agents, the most important diagnosis to exclude is an insulinoma, which is the most common cause of spontaneous, fasting hypoglycaemia in an otherwise healthy individual.

Insulinomas are benign tumours of pancreatic β-cells, with hypoglycaemia arising from excess secretion of insulin. The key investigation for insulinoma is a supervised fast, the premise of which is to elicit Whipple's triad, which is required for diagnosis. Whipple's triad requires (1) symptoms to be associated with fasting or exercise, (2) confirmation of hypoglycaemia during these episodes and (3) reversal of symptoms on administering glucose. In this case, all three criteria are met, and the inappropriately high levels of insulin at the end of the fast (with a glucose level of 1.8 mM) confirm hyperinsulinism. The high C-peptide levels confirm an endogenous rather than exogenous cause (C-peptide is the other product from cleavage of pro-insulin and is released with insulin from β-cells).

As the majority of insulinomas are single and benign, the treatment of choice is surgical resection. Further investigations are needed for tumour localisation, including abdominal ultrasound and CT; endoscopic ultrasound may be useful to identify pancreatic lesions. If these are not fruitful, selective angiography of pancreatic vessels with calcium stimulation (to cause vesicle release) and measurement of insulin levels in the hepatic vein may help locate the tumour anatomically.

While awaiting surgery, options to manage the hypoglycaemia include cornstarch infusion at night (this releases glucose in a slow, sustained fashion) and diazoxide, a thiazide-type drug that opens the K_{ATP} channel, leading to efflux of K^+ from β-cells, which causes hyperpolarisation and reduced insulin release.

The finding of an insulinoma in a young patient should raise the possibility of an endocrine syndrome, in particular multiple endocrine neoplasia type 1 (MEN1). This is an autosomal dominant syndrome characterised by tumours in the pancreas, pituitary and parathyroids ('3Ps') caused by germline mutations in the *MEN1* gene. While insulinoma is generally not a presenting feature of MEN1, the family history of 'thyroid problems' should serve to raise notice about its relevance to this patient.

 KEY POINTS

- The symptoms of hypoglycaemia arise from neuroglycopenia and autonomic hyper-reactivity.
- The most common cause of fasting hypoglycaemia in an otherwise healthy person is an insulinoma.
- The diagnosis of insulinoma is made by fulfilling Whipple's triad.

CASE 9: A MIDDLE-AGED WOMAN WITH JAUNDICE

A 53-year-old woman presents to a fast-track referral clinic with a 3-week history of jaundice and generalised fatigue. She also complains of generalised itch and malaise. On direct questioning, she confirms that her urine has become darker over the past month, but denies abdominal pain. She confesses to a weight loss of 3 kg in the past few months. She smokes 10 cigarettes a day, and there is no pertinent family history.

Examination

Scleral icterus and scratch marks over her skin are noted, but abdominal palpation is unremarkable. There is no lymphadenopathy.

🔍 INVESTIGATIONS

Haemoglobin	11.5
White cells	7.8
Platelets	350
U+E	Normal
Bilirubin	55
Alanine aminotransferase	96
Aspartate aminotransferase	85
Alkaline phosphatase	274
Gamma glutamyl transferase	211
Albumin	32
International normalised ratio	1.3

❓ QUESTIONS

1. Describe the metabolism of bilirubin.
2. What are the causes of jaundice, and how do the investigations help delineate between them?
3. Given the history, what is the most important diagnosis to exclude here, and how should the patient be further evaluated?

ANSWERS

The metabolism of bilirubin is summarised in Figure 9.1. In essence, bilirubin is a break-down product of haemoglobin and, as it is insoluble, it needs to be conjugated in the liver before it may be excreted. Some of the conjugated bilirubin is excreted in urine as urobilinogen (which is colourless) and in faeces as stercobilin (which is brown).

Hyperbilirubinaemia at levels >50 μM is sufficient to cause a yellowish discolouration of skin and sclerae (i.e. jaundice). The excess levels of bilirubin may either be conjugated or unconjugated depending on what part of the metabolic pathway is dysfunctional. There are five main causes of hyperbilirubinaemia: (1) excess production, (2) reduced hepatic uptake, (3) impaired conjugation, (4) reduced hepatocellular excretion and (5) impaired bile flow. Items 1, 2 and 3 produce an unconjugated hyperbilirubinaemia, whereas items 4 and 5 lead to conjugated hyperbilirubinaemia.

The causes of jaundice are classically three-fold:

1. Pre-hepatic. This causes an unconjugated hyperbilirubinaemia and arises from increased production of bilirubin (e.g., haemolysis, ineffective erythropoiesis).
2. Hepatic. The hyperbilirubinaemia may either be conjugated or unconjugated depending on which part of the hepatic metabolic pathway is affected. Congenital causes include Gilbert, Crigler-Najjar and Dubin-Johnson syndromes, while acquired causes include viral hepatitis, autoimmune hepatitis, alcoholic liver disease, drugs (e.g., halothane, paracetamol and methyldopa) and primary biliary cirrhosis.
3. Post-hepatic. This typically causes a conjugated hyperbilirubinaemia and arises as a result of biliary obstruction, causes of which include gallstones, malignancy (pancreatic cancer, cholangiocarcinoma and ampullary tumours of the duodenum), biliary strictures, pancreatic pseudocysts and sclerosing cholangitis.

The presence of dark urine in this case indicates a conjugated hyperbilirubinaemia arising from biliary obstruction. This colour is due to conjugated bilirubin, which leaks from hepatocytes or the biliary system when its excretory route is blocked and enters the systemic circulation, with some of it being excreted in urine. The pruritus arises from accumulation of bile salts in the skin, which again suggests a cholestatic picture.

The liver function results are suggestive of a post-hepatic cause, with proportionately greater elevation of ALP compared to AST or ALT. The latter two are liver-specific enzymes released from damaged hepatocytes and are raised in hepatocellular causes of jaundice. In contrast,

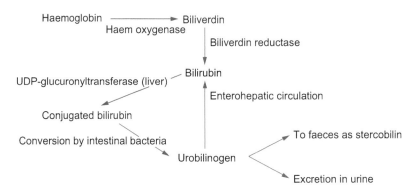

Figure 9.1 Metabolism of bilirubin.

ALP activity increases as a result of cholestasis stimulating greater enzyme synthesis. The elevation of INR may be due to vitamin K malabsorption, which is likely due to an obstruction causing bile salt deficiency (bile salts are needed for the absorption of the fat-soluble vitamins A, D, E and K).

A history of painless jaundice and constitutional symptoms with investigations favouring a post-hepatic picture should raise the suspicion of pancreatic carcinoma (or any other biliary malignancy). Further evaluation would begin with an abdominal ultrasound, which may identify any pancreatic lesions, as well as inform on the degree of biliary dilatation. Abdominal CT would be required to evaluate the pancreas and look for any metastases; if any lesions were found, a tissue diagnosis would be needed, most likely obtained by endoscopic ultrasound. It may also be worthwhile to measure tumour markers such as CA19–9 and carcinoembryonic antigen (CEA).

 KEY POINTS

- Bilirubin is a breakdown product of haemoglobin and is conjugated before being excreted by the liver.
- Jaundice occurs from elevated levels of bilirubin in the body, and its causes are conveniently categorised as pre-hepatic, hepatic or post-hepatic.
- Measurement of liver enzymes helps distinguish between the causes, with a disproportionately elevated ALP suggestive of biliary obstruction and high AST/ALT indicative of hepatocyte damage.

CASE 10: DRUG OVERDOSE

A 19-year-old student is found by her flatmate on a Monday morning minimally responsive. She notices a large amount of vomitus by the bedside and several packs of paracetamol tablets lying on the floor. At hospital, her friend informs the doctors that she last saw the patient on Saturday night after a big argument had taken place between the patient and her boyfriend. The patient confesses to taking numerous paracetamol tablets with alcohol throughout the day on Sunday, but is unable to recollect the precise number, though she informs the doctor that her last tablet was taken at 6 pm on the previous evening.

Examination

The patient is haemodynamically stable (T 37, HR 90, BP 110/65, O_2 sat 97% on room air). Abdominal examination reveals diffuse abdominal tenderness, most prominent in the right upper quadrant.

? QUESTIONS

1. What investigations are necessary for this patient?
2. What is the mechanism of paracetamol toxicity?
3. How should the patient be treated? Would management be affected if the patient were unable to remember when she last took the tablets?

DOI: 10.1201/9781003242697-11

ANSWERS

Paracetamol is the most common drug taken in overdose in the UK, with around 80,000 cases and 150–200 deaths each year. It is one of the leading causes of acute liver failure. The key aspects of dealing with a suspected paracetamol overdose are a thorough history, complete physical examination and prompt investigations. The aim of the history is to determine the quantity and chronology of the tablets taken, as well as to ascertain whether the patient has risk factors for hepatotoxicity (e.g., background liver disease, malnourishment, excess alcohol consumption, enzyme-inducing medication). Physical examination is directed mainly at evaluating for possible liver disease, while the key investigations that need to be performed are (1) urinalysis (for ketones), (2) timed serum paracetamol level, (3) liver function, (4) clotting screen (a marker of synthetic liver function) and (5) renal function.

The clinical features of paracetamol overdose are dependent on time. In the first 24 hours, patients may complain of nausea or vomiting, while serum transaminases may start to rise. One to two days post-overdose, abdominal signs and symptoms increase, with a continued rise in transaminases and possible evidence of liver dysfunction (coagulopathy). After this time, untreated patients may develop acute liver failure, with ensuing coagulopathy encephalopathy, and renal failure.

The recommended dosing of paracetamol is a maximum dose of 4 g a day for adults. Normally, the drug is metabolised by cytochrome P4502E1 to form a reactive metabolite, N-acetyl-p-benzoquinoneimine (NAPQI), which can be hepatotoxic. However, NAPQI is detoxified by glutathione, and hence, when there are sufficient amounts of the latter, the liver is not damaged. Overdoses of the drug deplete glutathione stores, and hepatic damage results. Glutathione stores also depend on nutritional status, which is why it is important to assess for background risk of liver damage.

The key investigation for paracetamol overdose is measurement of paracetamol concentration in the blood 4–16 hours post-dose. Levels taken before 4 hours are inaccurate due to incomplete absorption, while those taken after 16 hours may be falsely high due to the liver injury that may have occurred. If levels are higher than the treatment threshold, the patient requires treatment with three sequential intravenous infusions of acetylcysteine, which can replenish glutathione stores. Additionally, all suspected paracetamol overdose patients require fluid replacement. If paracetamol has been taken in the past hour, activated charcoal may be of use in limiting drug absorption. In cases where the timing of the paracetamol dose(s) is unknown, treatment with acetylcysteine should be started immediately in any patient who is at potential risk. If risk assessment is uncertain, the latest guidelines allow for treatment with acetylcysteine irrespective of the plasma paracetamol level.

> 🔑 **KEY POINTS**
>
> - The most common drug taken in overdose in the UK is paracetamol.
> - The mechanism of paracetamol toxicity is via depletion of glutathione stores, which helps detoxify NAPQI, a metabolite of the drug.
> - Paracetamol levels need to be measured between 4 and 16 hours after the last dose in order to decide whether treatment is required.

CASE 11: FATIGUE, WEAKNESS AND CONSTIPATION

A 60-year-old woman presents to her GP with several non-specific complaints. She has been suffering from generalised fatigue and muscle weakness for the past couple of months, as well as reduced frequency of bowel opening and 1.5 kg of weight loss. She has a past history of depression, hypertension and kidney stones.

Examination

Physical examination of her cardiovascular, respiratory and neurologic systems is unremarkable. Abdominal examination reveals mild generalised tenderness and possible faecal loading. The neck is supple and non-tender and there is no lymphadenopathy.

INVESTIGATIONS

Haemoglobin	11.5
White cells	6.7
Platelets	340
Sodium	134
Potassium	3.7
Urea	4.5
Creatinine	100
Bilirubin	10
Aspartate aminotransferase	30
Alkaline phosphatase	96
Corrected calcium	2.75
Thyroid-stimulating hormone	1.5

QUESTIONS

1. Suggest a differential diagnosis to account for her elevated serum calcium.
2. What additional investigations are required to further evaluate this patient?
3. If the cause is related to the parathyroid glands, how should the patient be managed and what would be the indications to intervene?

ANSWERS

Hypercalcaemia is the only abnormality in the blood tests and is frequently seen in primary care settings. It typically presents in a chronic setting, and the clinical features may be remembered via the 'renal stones, skeletal bones, abdominal moans, psychic groans' mnemonic.

There are several possible causes of hypercalcaemia:

- Hyperparathyroidism, which may be primary (e.g., parathyroid adenoma), secondary (from renal failure leading to hyperphosphataemia and stimulation of parathyroid hormone [PTH] secretion) or tertiary (autonomous parathyroid activity arising from secondary hyperparathyroidism)
- Malignancy associated, which may be either humorally mediated (e.g., release of parathyroid hormone-related protein [PTHrP] from squamous cell carcinomas) or osteolytic (e.g., multiple myeloma and bone metastases)
- Vitamin D–related (granulomatous diseases such as sarcoidosis, vitamin D excess)
- Drug-induced (e.g., thiazide diuretics)
- Endocrine disorders, including thyrotoxicosis
- Genetic disorders (e.g., familial hypocalciuric hypercalcaemia [FHH])

Of these, the first two are by far the most common causes, accounting for up to 90% of cases, and therefore require the closest attention when evaluating the patient.

Investigations to elucidate the underlying cause should be preceded by a careful history (including medications) and examination, with emphasis on examination of the neck (to assess the parathyroid glands) and searching for a possible tumour (e.g., chest and breast examination). A full blood count is required to look for possible evidence of chronic disease, renal function is needed to identify possible secondary hyperparathyroidism, and phosphate levels may be useful.

A key investigation is the measurement of serum PTH, with suppressed PTH levels indicating feedback inhibition from high calcium levels arising from an extra-parathyroid source (a likely malignancy). In this situation, investigation for malignancy (e.g., chest radiographs, mammogram and serum and urine electrophoresis for myeloma) would be warranted. High PTH levels would indicate primary (or tertiary) hyperparathyroidism, which may be confirmed with measurement of 24-hour urinary calcium. If these are unable to identify either malignancy or primary hyperparathyroidism, attention should be diverted towards the less common causes of hypercalcaemia.

Primary hyperparathyroidism is the most common cause of hypercalcaemia and typically affects older people, particularly women. Management of this condition is conservative (observation), medical (some evidence supports the use of bisphosphonates and cinacalcet, which inhibits PTH release), or surgical (via parathyroidectomy). A parathyroidectomy is recommended only for symptomatic patients or for asymptomatic individuals who are young (<50 years), have renal failure (estimated glomerular filtration rate [eGFR] <60), have reduced bone density (T score < −2.5 or previous fragility fracture) or whose serum calcium is 0.25 mM above the upper limit of normal.

🔑 **KEY POINTS**

- Hypercalcaemia usually presents in a vague fashion with several, seemingly unrelated complaints such as fatigue, constipation and polyuria.
- The two most common causes are hyperparathyroidism and malignancy related. Measurement of PTH helps distinguish between these.

CASE 12: EXCESSIVE HAIR GROWTH AND INFERTILITY

A 22-year-old woman presents to her GP because she is embarrassed by 'excessive hair growth' on her upper lip, lower abdomen and thighs. She has waxed her legs and body and shaved her upper lip weekly throughout her teenage years. On direct questioning, she reports that her periods have been irregular since menarche and that she is having difficulty conceiving despite regular unprotected sexual intercourse with her partner for the past year. Her family history is significant for diabetes and hypertension in her mother and maternal grandfather.

Examination

Physical examination reveals a mildly obese woman (body mass index [BMI] 31) with moderate facial acne and confirms hirsutism (Ferriman-Gallwey score 15). Examination of the genitalia is unremarkable, with a patent outflow tract and no clitoromegaly. Bimanual examination reveals a mobile anteverted uterus.

 INVESTIGATIONS

- FBC, renal profile: Normal
- Urine β-hCG: Negative

? QUESTIONS

1. Suggest a differential diagnosis for the cause of this woman's hirsutism.
2. Based on the clinical picture, what is the most likely diagnosis and why? What do you know about the aetiology of this condition?
3. What further investigations would be useful to confirm the likely diagnosis?
4. What are the management options in treating this woman's symptoms and overall condition?
5. Are there longer-term health problems that need to be considered in this patient?

DOI: 10.1201/9781003242697-13

ANSWERS

Medically, hirsutism refers to excessive terminal hair growth in a male pattern in women. Up to 5% of women of reproductive age are hirsute, according to the Ferriman-Gallwey scale (which scores hair growth in the most androgen-dependent parts of the body, with a score >7 defined as hirsute). As sexual hair growth is entirely androgen-dependent, androgen levels and the sensitivity of hair follicles to androgens are the primary factors leading to hirsutism. However, women with milder hirsutism may not show elevated androgen levels and have what is known as idiopathic hirsutism, which accounts for around 50% of cases. The remainder of cases are associated with hyperandrogenism, the causes of which are (1) polycystic ovarian syndrome (PCOS), (2) adrenogenital syndromes (e.g., non-classic congenital adrenal hyperplasia), (3) androgen-secreting tumours, (4) other causes of hormone overproduction such as Cushing's syndrome and (5) drug-induced.

In this woman, the main presenting complaints of hirsutism and difficulty conceiving, with probable anovulation, are consistent with a diagnosis of PCOS. PCOS affects up to 10% of women of reproductive age and is the underlying factor in around 15–20% of infertility cases. A diagnosis of PCOS, according to the 2003 Rotterdam PCOS Consensus Group, can be made with two of the following three findings: (1) clinical or biochemical evidence of androgen excess, (2) oligovulation or anovulation and (3) polycystic ovaries on ultrasound. The clinical findings in this case are sufficient to meet the first two of these, allowing a putative diagnosis of PCOS to be made.

While the exact pathophysiology of PCOS is unclear, one theory suggests that increased gonadotrophin-releasing hormone (GnRH) pulsing leads to increased luteinising hormone (LH) pulsing, stimulating increased production of androgens by theca cells in the ovary. There is also evidence that women with PCOS have elevated levels of insulin, which is known to act synergistically with LH to enhance androgen production by theca cells. Further, insulin inhibits synthesis of sex hormone–binding globulin (SHBG) by the liver, thereby increasing the proportion of free testosterone in the blood. These effects of insulin account for the hyperandrogenaemia in PCOS, which disrupts the normal follicular development process, leading to anovulation.

Before a diagnosis of PCOS can confidently be made, other conditions that produce hyperandrogenism and irregular menstrual cycles need to be excluded. Further investigations that may be performed to look for other causes include:

- Thyroid function (hypothyroidism)
- Serum prolactin (hyperprolactinaemia)
- 24-hour urinary cortisol (Cushing's syndrome)
- Morning 17-hydroxyprogesterone levels (elevated in non-classic congenital adrenal hyperplasia)
- Oral glucose tolerance test and growth hormone suppression (acromegaly)
- Follicle-stimulating hormone (FSH) and oestradiol (high and low/normal, respectively, in premature ovarian failure)

Biochemical investigations may show increased testosterone levels, reduced SHBG, increased LH and a high LH:FSH ratio. An ovarian ultrasound should be performed to visualise the ovaries.

Management of PCOS is essentially symptomatic. Hirsutism and acne are managed by agents designed to inhibit hyperandrogenism, such as the combined oral contraceptive pill, anti-androgens (such as cyproterone acetate or spironolactone), and eflornithine hydrochloride, as well as laser or electrolysis for hair removal. The presence of chronic anovulation carries a higher risk of endometrial hyperplasia and carcinoma, and therefore requires treatment (typically with the contraceptive pill or cyclical progestogens). Ovulation may be induced with the use of clomiphene (an oestrogen receptor antagonist at the hypothalamus).

PCOS also carries a significant risk for the development of metabolic and cardiovascular disease, including obesity, impaired glucose tolerance and diabetes and accelerated atherosclerosis. The likely pathophysiology behind these is insulin resistance, since women with PCOS are usually hyperinsulinaemic. These longer-term complications require similar management to type 2 diabetes, with weight reduction and certain antidiabetic agents (metformin and the thiazolidinediones) forming the mainstay of treatment.

 KEY POINTS

- Hirsutism refers to the excessive growth of hair in a male pattern in women.
- It may arise from elevated androgen levels or be idiopathic.
- PCOS is a clinical diagnosis that often presents with hirsutism and oligomenorrhea or amenorrhoea.
- The mechanism of hyperandrogenism in PCOS is unclear but may relate to increased GnRH and LH pulsing.

CASE 13: FATIGUE AND IRREGULAR PERIODS

A 50-year-old female pilot undergoes a medical screening examination prior to joining a new airline. She has been generally fit and well over the past few months. She reports some tiredness, but "nothing that a good holiday would not solve". She has a past history of a ductal carcinoma of the breast, which was excised and has completed 10-year follow-up without any concerns. Her periods are becoming increasingly irregular, and she has noticed a few hot flushes recently.

Examination

Physical examination reveals a well-looking, slightly overweight woman. There is slight fullness in the anterior neck that is smooth, regular and non-tender, compatible with a goitre. There is no associated lymphadenopathy.

INVESTIGATIONS

Haemoglobin	11.9
White cells	6.7
Platelets	245
Sodium	137
Potassium	4.2
Urea	4.5
Creatinine	75
Thyroid-stimulating hormone	8
Free T4	11
Thyroid autoAb	+ve (anti-TPO)

QUESTIONS

1. What are the possible causes of a goitre?
2. Interpret the thyroid function test result. What thyroid state is suggested by these values, and what common causes may account for them?
3. Is any treatment required for this patient?

ANSWERS

A goitre refers to an enlarged thyroid gland and is one of the most common causes of a mass in the muscular triangle of the neck. The basic pathophysiology of a goitre is stimulation of thyroid follicular cells by thyroid-stimulating hormone (TSH). Therefore, causes of goitre include any cause of hypothyroidism (e.g., iodine deficiency, thyroiditis, TSH-secreting pituitary tumours, thyroid dyshormogenesis and thyroid hormone resistance). Autoantibodies stimulating the TSH receptor also produce a goitre, as seen in Graves' disease. Certain substances (e.g., amiodarone, cassava) can interfere with iodine uptake by the thyroid and can therefore cause increased TSH secretion and subsequent goitre. Additional causes of thyroid enlargement include tumours (benign adenomas or malignant carcinomas), infection and granulomatous diseases.

This woman's blood results are normal except for thyroid function. TSH is elevated at twice the upper limit of normal, but free T4 levels are within the normal range. These results could be consistent with two possibilities:

1. Subclinical or compensated hypothyroidism
2. Treated hyperthyroidism

The absence of any history of thyroid disease makes subclinical hypothyroidism the likeliest diagnosis. This indicates some degree of thyroid failure that is partly compensated for by a rise in TSH levels, which is sufficient to keep thyroxine levels in the normal range. There are typically only non-specific or very mild symptoms in this condition.

Subclinical hypothyroidism is frequently associated with anti-thyroid antibodies (e.g., anti-TPO), which is a marker of Hashimoto's thyroiditis, an autoimmune thyroid disease that affects up to 2% of the population. Other causes of subclinical hypothyroidism include partial thyroidectomy, radioiodide treatment, external radiotherapy to the neck, infiltrative disorders affecting the thyroid gland (e.g., amyloidosis, sarcoidosis) and inadequate thyroxine replacement for hypothyroidism. Given the demographics of the patient and positivity to anti-TPO, Hashimoto's thyroiditis is the most likely diagnosis in this patient.

Subclinical hypothyroidism may progress to overt thyroid failure, but also has other physiologic effects, including impairment of cardiac function and increasing low-density lipoprotein (LDL) cholesterol levels, both of which are responsible for the higher cardiovascular risk seen in patients.

Treatment with thyroxine replacement for subclinical hypothyroidism is controversial. Various factors, including age and background cardiovascular risk status, symptomatology (e.g., goitre), antibody positivity and TSH levels, need to be considered before making a decision on whether to commence treatment. In this case, antibody positivity suggests an autoimmune thyroid disease that will likely progress to overt hypothyroidism. Given the additional finding of a goitre, it would likely be prudent to begin thyroxine replacement.

🔑 KEY POINTS

- A thyroid goitre arises through excess stimulation of thyroid follicular cells by TSH.
- Subclinical hypothyroidism is frequently encountered and may progress to overt thyroid failure, particularly if autoantibodies are positive, indicating the likelihood of Hashimoto's thyroiditis.
- There is no consensus on whether subclinical hypothyroidism should always be treated, though it is worth remembering that the condition carries an increased cardiovascular risk.

CASE 14: STIFF AND PAINFUL HANDS

A 28-year-old legal assistant presents to her GP after being bothered by stiffness in the joints of both of her hands for the past few weeks. The stiffness is most prominent on awakening and lasts approximately an hour before getting better through the day. She denies any other musculoskeletal problems or any other joints being affected. Her only medical history is mild asthma. Her family history is positive for type 1 diabetes in her brother.

Examination

Physical examination reveals a well-looking, slim woman. Her metacarpophalangeal joints are slightly swollen bilaterally and mildly tender, and there is some pain on palpation over a few of the interphalangeal joints in both hands. Metacarpal squeeze test is positive bilaterally.

? QUESTIONS

1. Based on the history and examination findings, suggest a differential diagnosis. Which diagnosis is most likely and why?
2. What further investigations are required, and which tests are most predictive for the likely diagnosis?
3. Summarise the pathophysiology of the underlying diagnosis. What extra-articular complications may arise with this condition?

ANSWERS

The clinical picture in this case is very suggestive of an inflammatory arthropathy with the findings of joint swelling, morning stiffness and evidence of synovitis. The key differential diagnoses therefore include:

- Rheumatoid arthritis (RA)
- Seronegative spondyloarthropathies (e.g., psoriatic arthritis, arthritis associated with inflammatory bowel disease)
- Post-viral or post-infectious arthropathy
- Connective tissue diseases (such as lupus and scleroderma)
- Crystal arthropathy (gout and pseudogout)
- Degenerative joint disease (osteoarthritis)

The most likely diagnosis is RA, which is the most common inflammatory arthropathy and typically affects adults between the ages of 30 and 50. This is because the history of bilateral joint problems, mainly in the small joints of the hand, as well as morning stiffness lasting longer than 1 hour, is very suggestive of an inflammatory rather than a degenerative process (in the latter, symptoms tend to get worse throughout the day, and stiffness generally lasts less than an hour). Similarly, the absence of any background medical history or other symptoms makes seronegative arthritis, post-viral arthritis and connective tissue disease unlikely.

The diagnosis of RA requires the following, based on American College of Rheumatology/ European Alliance of Associations for Rheumatology (ACR/EULAR) criteria:

- Inflammatory arthritis involving three or more joint areas
- Seropositivity for rheumatoid factor or anti–citrullinated protein (CCP)
- Elevated levels of inflammatory markers (ESR or CRP)
- Exclusion of other diseases such as crystal arthropathy, post-viral arthropathy, psoriatic arthritis and lupus
- Duration of symptoms lasting >6 weeks

This patient meets three of these criteria from history and examination alone, and referral to a rheumatology specialist would be warranted. Further investigations would include basic blood tests (full blood count—possible anaemia of chronic disease, renal and hepatic function—which may guide medication choice) and tests of inflammatory activity. The latter include CRP and ESR along with more specific tests for RA, namely rheumatoid factor (RF) and anti-CCP antibodies. Anti-CCP has a similar sensitivity (65–85%) but much higher specificity (>95% vs. 80%) for RA in patients with suspected rheumatic disease than RF, and anti-CCP positivity is also associated with a more severe clinical course. Radiographs of the hand would also be useful to look for evidence of joint damage.

The pathophysiology of RA is incompletely understood, and the cause remains unknown. It is an autoimmune disease triggered by the exposure of a genetically susceptible individual to an as-yet unidentified antigen. Interplay of genetic (e.g., human leukocyte antigen [HLA]-DR4 allele) and environmental (e.g., smoking, infection) factors lead to altered post-transcriptional regulation of proteins and citrullination of self-proteins. Loss of tolerance to these new epitopes leads to the formation of autoantibodies (e.g., anti-CCP) and the stimulation of B-cell and CD4 T-cell responses, which act against unknown target antigens in joints and mediate joint injury via production of inflammatory cytokines such as tumour necrosis factor alpha (TNF-α) and interleukin (IL)-1. These stimulate proliferation of synovial cells and the production of matrix metalloproteinases, which assist in the destruction of articular cartilage, and the inflammatory-rich hyperplastic synovium adheres to and grows over the articular surfaces, forming pannus.

RA is also associated with an increased risk of cardiovascular disease, resulting from endothelial activation by inflammatory cytokines. This generalised inflammatory response may also account for the other systemic manifestations of RA, involving the lungs (fibrosis), bones (osteoporosis) and brain (reduced cognition), as well as a higher risk of lymphoma.

🔑 KEY POINTS

- Morning stiffness is a common rheumatologic symptom, and the key to distinguishing whether it is inflammatory or degenerative in origin is seeing whether it gets better or worse through the day.
- RA typically affects the small joints of the hands bilaterally and is associated with positivity for anti-CCP antibodies.
- It is believed to arise from the immune system reacting against as-yet unidentified antigens, provoking the formation of an inflammatory pannus over articular surfaces.

CASE 15: ABDOMINAL PAIN, NAUSEA AND VOMITING

A 15-year-old boy is brought into the emergency department after complaining of abdominal pain throughout the day. He has been feeling generally unwell for the past couple of days, but is much worse today with a decline in his level of alertness. He is drowsy but still communicates in sentences and complains of a productive cough. He has had three episodes of non-bilious, non-bloody vomiting over the past few hours and gives a vague history of drinking more water in the past few weeks. His past medical history is significant for asthma.

Examination

Physical examination reveals an ill-looking boy with pulse of 100, blood pressure 110/70 mmHg, respiratory rate 24 per minute and shallow, O_2 saturation of 95% on room air, temperature 35.8°C and Glasgow Coma Scale (GCS) 14 (E4, V4, M6). Auscultation of the chest is positive for crackles at the right mid and lower zones. Abdominal palpation reveals a diffusely tender abdomen, but no guarding or rebound tenderness. No focal neurology is demonstrable.

INVESTIGATIONS

Haemoglobin	13.6
White cells	13
Neutrophils	8
Platelets	340
Sodium	138
Potassium	5.2
Chloride	105
Urea	10.9
Creatinine	90
Bilirubin	10
Alkaline phosphatase	56
C-reactive protein	125
Glucose	22.5

Urine dipstick +++ glucose and ketones

ABG (on room air):

pH	7.30
pCO_2	12.1
pCO_2	3.5
HCO_3	17

? QUESTIONS

1. Interpret the arterial blood gas results. What type of disorder is suggested?
2. What are the potential causes of this metabolic disturbance? Which is the likeliest cause (given the history and examination)?
3. Discuss the pathophysiology underlying the likely condition. What is the likely precipitant?
4. What are the principles of managing this patient in the short term?

ANSWERS

The arterial blood gas is consistent with a partly compensated metabolic acidosis. The low pH and the low bicarbonate levels confirm that the cause of the acidosis is metabolic; since pCO_2 is slightly low, there is some degree of respiratory compensation in an effort to blow off H^+ as CO_2. This correlates with the clinical finding of a high respiratory rate and shallow breathing (Kussmaul's breathing).

When investigating a metabolic acidosis, it is useful to determine the anion gap ($[Na^+]$ + $[K^+] - [Cl^-] - [HCO_3^-]$), as the causes of a normal anion-gap metabolic acidosis are distinct from those of a raised anion-gap acidosis. Here, the anion gap is 21, which is elevated, indicating that an unmeasured anion is present in increased quantities (such as lactate, β-hydroxybutyrate). The causes of a metabolic acidosis with a high anion gap include:

- Lactic acidosis (e.g., tissue hypoxia, drugs such as metformin and ethanol)
- Ketoacidosis (e.g., diabetic ketoacidosis)
- Exogenous acids (e.g., salicylate overdose)
- Accumulation of organic acids (e.g., inherited organic acidoses)
- Renal failure ('uraemic acidosis')

Here, the likeliest cause is diabetic ketoacidosis (DKA), given the symptoms of abdominal pain and vomiting on a background of feeling generally unwell with polyuria. The finding of Kussmaul's breathing is also characteristic. Additionally, blood tests confirm hyperglycaemia, with the presence of both glucose and ketones in urine.

DKA is a medical emergency, accounting for up to 10% of hospital admissions for children with diabetes. It can often be the first manifestation of a previously undiagnosed case of type 1 diabetes and comprises three key elements: (1) marked hyperglycaemia, (2) ketosis and (3) acidosis. It results from acute insulin deficiency, which leads to the following:

- Rapid mobilisation of energy from muscle and fat stores, with conversion of amino acids to glucose and fatty acids to ketones
- The low insulin:glucagon ratio and higher levels of catecholamines and cortisol promoting hepatic glycogenolysis and gluconeogenesis
- Reduced peripheral utilisation of glucose and ketones due to lack of insulin, thereby leading to hyperglycaemia and ketosis
- Hyperglycaemia provoking an osmotic diuresis, leading to depletion of intravascular volume, with reduction in renal blood flow hampering the ability of the kidneys to excrete glucose, and resultant hyperosmolality, which may lead to central nervous system (CNS) depression and coma

The precipitating factor here is probably a chest infection. The stress response to infection invokes a counter-regulatory hormone drive, with a rise in the glucagon:insulin ratio, leading to the sequence of events described above.

The key aspects of managing DKA are four-fold:

- Immediate resuscitation
- Fluid and electrolyte replacement
- Insulin replacement
- Treatment of precipitating causes

Emergency management should follow an ABCDE approach and be combined with fluid resuscitation. At least 2 L of normal saline are required in adult patients in the first 2–3 hours to reduce the hyperosmolar state, clear ketones and restore extracellular fluid volume. The overall fluid deficit in an average adult may be up to 7 L. As soon as fluid resuscitation is under way, insulin replacement by way of a fixed-rate insulin infusion (0.1 units/kg) is required. The aim should be to reduce blood ketone concentrations by at least 0.5 mM per hour and capillary blood glucose by 3 mM per hour and to raise venous bicarbonate by 3 mM per hour. Once blood glucose levels fall below 14 mM, 10% glucose infusion is recommended to avoid hypoglycaemia, with continuation of the insulin infusion to suppress ketogenesis.

The electrolyte deficiencies in DKA include sodium, potassium, chloride and phosphate. Potassium losses may be particularly high (though serum levels may be artificially high from the potassium flux into the extracellular space as a result of acidosis), and generally 40 mmol of K^+ is given with each bag of normal saline. In addition to these resuscitative measures, treatment should be directed at the precipitating cause (e.g., antibiotics for chest infection), and the diabetic specialist team should be involved in management, particularly as they will be needed to plan long-term treatment.

 KEY POINTS

- Calculation of the anion gap helps distinguish between the causes of a metabolic acidosis.
- DKA is a common cause of a raised anion-gap metabolic acidosis and fundamentally results from acute insulin deficiency.
- Management of DKA is based on replacing the deficient insulin, fluid and electrolytes and treating the provoking cause.

CASE 16: FREQUENT THROAT AND CHEST INFECTIONS

A 28-year-old woman presents to her GP with a chesty cough that has been ongoing for 4 days and is now productive of green sputum. This is her fourth such episode this year. She says that she has suffered from 'sinus infections' since she was a teenager. She has a history of asthma as well as intermittent abdominal pain and diarrhoea that began after a holiday to South America.

Examination

Vital signs are T 37.6°C, HR 90, BP 110/65, RR 22, O$_2$ sat 96% on room air. Physical examination reveals crackles in the right mid and lower lung zones.

INVESTIGATIONS

Haemoglobin	11.5
White cells	11.5
Platelets	225
IgG	Low
IgA	Undetectable
IgM	Normal
HIV antigen	Negative

QUESTIONS

1. What initial screening tests should be performed if her physician suspects an immunodeficiency?
2. Assuming there are no secondary causes, what would be the most likely cause of a primary immunodeficiency in this woman? What do you know about the aetiology of this condition?
3. How should this woman be managed for the likely underlying condition? What other complications need to be monitored for?

ANSWERS

Immunodeficiency should be suspected in patients with severe, persistent, recurrent, or 'unusual' infections; in this case, the history of recurrent sinopulmonary infections is suspicious, while the presence of chronic diarrhoea should also raise the suspicion of an infectious gastroenteritis (e.g., giardiasis).

Immunodeficiency may be either primary (an intrinsic immune system defect) or secondary to an underlying condition. Important secondary causes of immunodeficiency to consider are infections (notably HIV), malnutrition, malignancy (particularly haematologic), drugs (immunosuppressants, immunomodulators), protein-losing states (e.g., nephrotic syndrome, protein-losing enteropathy) and metabolic disease (e.g., diabetes and severe liver disease).

Initial workup of a suspected immunodeficiency involves taking a pertinent history and performing a complete examination. Investigations should include a full blood count, liver and renal function tests, urinalysis (for proteinuria), HIV status, measurement of total serum proteins and relevant imaging for sinusitis and chest infections. Measurement of serum immunoglobulins is crucial to look for antibody deficiencies.

Here, serum immunoglobulin levels show low levels of IgG and IgA with normal IgM levels. If secondary causes are ruled out, the key causes of primary immunodeficiency to consider are (1) common variable immunodeficiency (CVID), (2) X-linked agammaglobulinaemia (XLA), (3) selective Ig subclass deficiency and (4) hyper-IgM syndrome. All cause antibody deficiency, but XLA presents in the neonatal period, while levels of IgM are greatly increased in hyper-IgM syndrome. Selective Ig deficiency may be a possibility here, but is less likely given that two different immunoglobulins are deficient. Hence, the most likely diagnosis, partly by exclusion and partly because of the age of the patient, is CVID.

CVID, the most common symptomatic primary immunodeficiency, typically presents in late childhood with recurrent sinopulmonary and bacterial infections as well as gastrointestinal complications. Capsulated bacteria (*Haemophilus influenzae* and *Streptococcus pneumoniae*) account for the bulk of respiratory infections, while *Giardia* is more frequent given the deficiency in mucosal antibody defences.

CVID is usually sporadic, and though the molecular basis of the disease is incompletely understood, the defect lies in the inability of B cells in blood and lymphoid tissue (present in normal numbers) to differentiate into plasma cells. It is unclear whether this is an intrinsic B-cell problem or whether the fault lies with a defective ability of T cells in activating B cells.

The mainstay of CVID management is immunoglobulin replacement and prompt treatment of infections. Further, attention should be paid to potential complications of CVID, which include an increased risk of autoimmune disease (e.g., haemolytic anaemia), lung disease (e.g., bronchiectasis, fibrosis), granulomatous disease (usually affecting the lung) and cancer (particularly lymphoid malignancy).

🔑 **KEY POINTS**

- Suspect an immunodeficiency if there is evidence of severe, persistent, recurrent or unusual infections.
- Immunodeficiency may be either primary or secondary to an underlying condition such as HIV.
- CVID is the most common symptomatic primary immunodeficiency and is due to a defect in differentiation of B cells into antibody-secreting plasma cells.

CASE 17: A ROUTINE 'HEALTH CHECK' FOR A 55-YEAR-OLD MAN

A 55-year-old man presents to his GP for his annual check-up. He has a history of hypertension, which is controlled by amlodipine, and hyperlipidaemia, for which he takes a statin. He does not complain of any particular symptoms, but notes that he has been urinating more frequently. He wonders whether this may be an early sign of diabetes, as both his brothers have recently been diagnosed with this condition. He has a family history of cardiovascular disease, with both his parents having suffered a heart attack in their 60s. He recently stopped smoking but has a 35 pack-year history.

Examination

Body mass index (BMI) is 28. Cardiovascular, respiratory, abdominal and neurologic examinations are unremarkable. Digital rectal examination reveals a small and benign-feeling prostate.

? | **QUESTIONS**

1. What investigations may be used to diagnose diabetes in this gentleman?
2. Describe the pathophysiology of type 2 diabetes.
3. What are the complications of diabetes, and what do you know about their aetiology?
4. Discuss the overall principles of management of this patient, assuming he is found to be diabetic.

ANSWERS

Type 2 diabetes mellitus is predominantly a disease of the older population and accounts for 90% of cases of diabetes. It may be diagnosed through three tests: (1) fasting glucose levels, (2) glucose tolerance test and (3) glycated haemoglobin levels. Additionally, in this case, testing the urine for glucose might be useful, though it must be remembered that around 10% of cases of glycosuria are not caused by hyperglycaemia.

Fasting glucose levels were the easiest way in which to test for diabetes until glycated haemoglobin (HbA1c) assays became available. The World Health Organization (WHO) criteria for diabetes require a fasting glucose level of ≥7 mM, since that is the level above which the microvascular complications of diabetes become detectable. An oral glucose tolerance test (measuring plasma glucose 2 hours after a standardised glucose load, with levels ≥11.1 mM being diagnostic of diabetes) is a more sensitive marker of glucose dysregulation but is more expensive and less reproducible. More recently, the use of HbA1c levels have been used in diagnosing type 2 diabetes. HbA1c measures the non-enzymatic glycation of amino acids on the haemoglobin molecule and reflects the glycaemic state over the prior 8–12 weeks. Normal levels are between 4% and 6%, with the WHO recognising a threshold of 6.5% as the cut-off point for diagnosing type 2 diabetes.

The two main metabolic defects that underlie type 2 diabetes are insulin resistance and subsequent pancreatic β-cell dysfunction. The former is caused by both quantitative and qualitative changes in insulin signalling, such as reduced receptor tyrosine kinase activity, which is strongly linked to obesity ('lipotoxicity'). Initially, insulin resistance is compensated for by pancreatic β-cell hypersecretion of insulin; however, there is eventual decompensation, the mechanisms of which remain unclear, but are likely linked to lipotoxicity and 'glucotoxicity'. It is also important to be aware of the genetic link in type 2 diabetes, which is stronger than in type 1 diabetes.

Life expectancy in diabetics is reduced by 5–10 years compared to non-diabetics. The major causes of excess mortality are cardiovascular disease, renal problems and infection. Hence, the complications of diabetes are just as important to monitor as glycaemic control itself. Broadly speaking, these complications may be categorised as either microvascular (disease of small blood vessels) or macrovascular (large-vessel disease). Microvascular complications include retinopathy, nephropathy and neuropathy, while the predominant macrovascular complications are cardiovascular, cerebrovascular and peripheral vascular disease.

The principal mechanism underlying macrovascular complications is accelerated atherosclerosis of large vessels, leading to a higher risk of thrombosis and occlusion, while the basic pathophysiology underlying microangiopathy is thickening of capillary basement membranes in the retina, kidneys and vaso nervorum. In the kidney, these thickened capillaries are more leaky than normal to plasma proteins, giving rise to microalbuminuria. Similarly, in the eyes, microangiopathy gives rise to non-proliferative or proliferative retinopathy. Indeed, diabetes is the most common cause of blindness in individuals under 65 years of age.

Given the burden of disease that diabetes imposes, its management is multi-faceted. Patient education and dietary measures form the basis of conservative management, particularly in diabetics whose β-cells are able to compensate. Oral anti-diabetic agents that aim to either stimulate insulin secretion (e.g., sulphonylureas) or increase insulin sensitivity (e.g., metformin) may be required to optimise glycaemic control, and the last resort is insulin. However, it is important to remember that diabetes management is not just about controlling sugar levels but that hypertension and hyperlipidaemia need to be aggressively managed too. Additionally, patients with nephropathy require angiotensin-converting enzyme (ACE) inhibitors or angiotensin receptor antagonist therapy and regular diabetic eye screening is needed to monitor for retinopathy.

🔑 KEY POINTS

- Type 2 diabetes is the most common form of diabetes and may be diagnosed via measurement of fasting glucose levels, an oral glucose tolerance test, or HbA1c levels.
- The pathophysiology underlying the disease stems from insulin resistance and eventual pancreatic β-cell dysfunction and decompensation.
- Management of type 2 diabetes involves not only aggressive glycaemic control but also minimising cardiovascular risk factors and possible renal and retinal disease.

CASE 18: COLLAPSE IN A PATIENT UNDERGOING CHEMOTHERAPY

A 30-year-old man undergoing his first cycle of Adriamycin, bleomycin, vinblastine, dacarbazine (ABVD) chemotherapy for bulky stage II Hodgkin's lymphoma is brought into hospital by his wife after collapsing at home. His wife says that the patient has been vomiting several times over the past 24 hours and has been complaining of increased fatigue. Though drowsy, he says that he has been experiencing numbness in his hands over the past couple of hours as well.

Examination

Physical examination reveals an ill-looking man, with cool peripheries. His vital signs show T 36.2°C, BP 95/60, HR 100 and regular, RR 24 and 95% O_2 saturation on room air. An ECG shows peaked T waves and prolongation of the QRS (0.14 ms). A fingerprick glucose is 5.6 mM, and capillary refill time is 3 s. Glasgow Coma Scale (GCS) is 14/15 (E4, V4, M6).

Given his clinical state, the patient is catheterised, and urine output is 10 mL in the first 30 minutes, improving to 25 mL over the next 30 minutes after fluid resuscitation.

INVESTIGATIONS

Haemoglobin	11.9
White cells	5.6
Platelets	180
Sodium	133
Potassium	6.3
Urea	15.9
Creatinine	156
Bilirubin	10
Alanine aminotransferase	25
Aspartate aminotransferase	30
Alkaline phosphatase	110
Corrected calcium	1.65
Phosphate	1.8
International normalised ratio	1.1

? QUESTIONS

1. Renal function is grossly deranged in this patient. What are the possible causes of this, and how may they be differentiated?
2. Given the clinical picture and test results, suggest an underlying aetiology for this patient's presentation.
3. Discuss the pathophysiology of the likely underlying diagnosis.
4. What are the main aspects in managing this patient in the acute setting?

ANSWERS

This patient has acute renal failure, which may be defined as the rapid loss of renal function with retention of urea, creatinine and other metabolic products and usually characterised by oliguria. His urea and creatinine levels are around 1.5 times the upper limit of normal, while his urine output (prior to fluid resuscitation) of 20 mL/hr is significantly less than expected of an adult male. Classically, the causes of acute renal failure are categorised as:

- Pre-renal, which arises from hypovolaemia leading to inadequate renal blood flow (haemorrhage, sepsis, heart failure, diarrhoea and use of diuretics)
- Intrinsic renal disease, which may affect the glomeruli (e.g., various glomerulo-nephritides), tubules, and interstitium (e.g., drugs such as non-steroidal anti-inflammatory drugs [NSAIDs] and aminoglycosides, contrast media, and intrarenal obstruction arising from renal calculi or the cast nephropathy in multiple myeloma), or the blood vessels (e.g., vasculitis, hypertension, diabetes)
- Post-renal obstruction, which leads to renal failure when both outflow tracts are obstructed or when one is obstructed in patients with a single kidney (e.g., bladder outflow obstruction, ureteric calculi, intratubular crystal nephropathy, and urothelial neoplasms)

Measurement of urine composition and using ratios of serum urea:creatinine may help differentiate between the above when the history is not especially suggestive, as shown below.

Measure	Pre-renal	Renal	Post-renal
Urine osmolality (mOsm/kg)	>500	<350	<350
Urine Na (mM)	<10	>20	>40
Fractional excretion of Na (%)	<1	>2	>4
Serum Ur:Cr	>100:1	<40:1	40–100:1

Here, renal failure is accompanied by hyperkalaemia, hypocalcaemia and hyperphosphataemia. These are suggestive of tumour lysis syndrome (TLS) as the underlying aetiology for the renal failure, with hypovolaemia as a contributory factor too. TLS is classified as either laboratory TLS or clinical TLS. Laboratory TLS requires the presence of two or more metabolic abnormalities (hyperuricaemia, hyperkalaemia, hypocalcaemia, hyperphosphataemia) occurring 3 days prior to or up to 7 days after the start of anti-cancer therapy, whereas clinical TLS is present when laboratory TLS is accompanied by the clinical findings of raised serum creatinine, seizures, arrhythmia, or death. Our patient meets the criteria for both.

TLS is most frequently seen with chemotherapy against rapidly proliferating tumours, typically haematologic cancers, given their high rate of cell turnover. The pathophysiology behind TLS is the release of potassium, phosphorus and nucleic acids from rapidly dividing cancer cells when they begin to be lysed by anti-cancer therapy. Hyperphosphataemia gives rise to hypocalcaemia, and nucleic acids are metabolised to uric acid, producing hyperuricaemia. Renal failure may arise since both urate and phosphate can crystallise and cause intratubular obstruction. Crystal-independent mechanisms, including renal vasoconstriction and reduced renal blood flow, may also have a part to play. In this case, we see the manifestations of these metabolic abnormalities, with ECG changes suggestive of hyperkalaemia, paraesthesia probably induced by hypocalcaemia, and oliguria indicative of renal failure.

Given the patient's hypovolaemic state, which predisposes the patient to develop renal failure, the immediate management priority is fluid resuscitation. Hydration also helps minimise acidosis and increases urine pH, which reduces the risk of urate crystallisation. Hyperkalaemia requires intervention with calcium gluconate, insulin and dextrose, given that ECG changes are seen with the higher risk of arrhythmia. The other metabolic abnormality that requires urgent intervention is hyperuricaemia. Rasburicase, which converts uric acid to the inactive and soluble metabolite allantoin, may be preferred to xanthine oxidase inhibitors such as allopurinol, as rasburicase also breaks down existing uric acid, whereas allopurinol only prevents its further formation. Clinical TLS patients also often require management in an ITU setting, given the need for cardiac monitoring and supportive management of renal failure through haemofiltration.

🔑 KEY POINTS

- Acute renal failure is the rapid loss of renal function with retention of waste metabolites such as urea and creatinine and may be due to pre-renal, renal, or post-renal causes.
- TLS occurs with rapid lysis of rapidly proliferating cancer cells after anti-cancer therapy and produces several metabolic derangements, including hyperphosphataemia, hyperkalaemia and hyperuricaemia.
- Crystallisation of phosphate and urate may occlude renal tubules, causing renal failure.

CASE 19: A 10-DAY-OLD BABY WITH AMBIGUOUS GENITALIA

A 24-year-old refugee brings her 10-day-old child to hospital after finding the child less responsive than normal, not feeding appropriately and vomiting several times for the past few days. The baby was delivered vaginally at term by the child's aunt, and the mother received no pre- or post-natal care.

Examination

Examination reveals an ill-looking neonate with evidence of dehydration (HR 180, BP 65/30, CRT 3 s, sunken fontanelles). There are no rashes. On unclothing the child and examining the external genitalia, a phallic-appearing structure is noted and there is fusion of the skin folds surrounding it. No testes are palpated, and the physician is uncertain about the sex of the neonate.

INVESTIGATIONS

	Haemoglobin	17
	Haematocrit	55%
	White cells	14
	Sodium	135
	Potassium	6.2
	Urea	19.5
	Creatinine	65
ABG (on room air):		
	pH	7.28

QUESTIONS

1. What are the possible causes of ambiguous genitalia? What are the basic principles of evaluating this condition?
2. What is the likely diagnosis in this case and why?
3. What treatment does this baby now require?

ANSWERS

Around 1 in 4500 newborns have what may be considered 'ambiguous genitalia'. Broadly, there are two causal categories of ambiguous genitalia:

1. Virilised XX female. This may be the result of androgens of fetal origin (e.g., congenital adrenal hyperplasia [CAH]) or maternal (e.g., drugs such as progesterone and danazol, maternal androgen-secreting tumours of the ovary or adrenal gland). The other main causes are dysmorphic conditions such as Beckwith-Wiedemann and Seckel syndromes.
2. Undervirilised XY male. This may arise from a biosynthetic defect leading to reduced fetal androgen production (e.g., Leydig cell defects, 5-α-reductase deficiency, deficiency of anti-Mullerian hormone), end-organ unresponsiveness to androgens (androgen insensitivity syndrome), dysmorphic syndromes (e.g., Smith-Lemli-Opitz syndrome) and testicular dysgenesis or malfunction.

The evaluation of ambiguous genitalia should begin with the history to look for the use of any drugs that may cause female virilisation, any evidence of maternal virilisation that may suggest a maternal androgen-secreting tumour, and any family history of a genetic disorder. A complete examination of the child is required to assess its general condition, identify dysmorphic features, and assess the external genitalia (number of gonads, degree of virilisation, length of the phallus and any hyperpigmentation that would suggest excessive adrenocorticotropic hormone [ACTH] production). The most important initial tests are to determine karyotype and assess internal anatomy by way of pelvic ultrasound. The other priority is to avoid a salt-losing crisis (seen in CAH); therefore, blood tests for electrolytes, luteinising hormone (LH), follicle-stimulating hormone (FSH) and androgen levels (testosterone, dehydroepiandrosterone [DHEA], androstenedione and 17-OH-progestrone) are required.

In this neonate, physical examination is consistent with clitoromegaly and labial fusion, suggesting a virilised XX female, though formal karyotypical analysis is needed for confirmation. The blood tests are informative of the diagnosis, as they reveal mild hyponatraemia, hyperkalaemia, evidence of hypovolaemia and acidosis. These are consistent with the salt-wasting form of 21-hydroxylase deficiency, the enzyme defect accounting for more than 90% of cases of CAH.

CAH is an autosomal recessive condition caused by deficiencies of one of five enzymes required for adrenal steroid synthesis (see Figure 19.1). 21-Hydroxylase is required for the synthesis of aldosterone and cortisol but not that of adrenal androgens. Deficiency of cortisol leads to feedback upregulation of ACTH, which overstimulates the adrenal cortex, producing adrenal hyperplasia. Since a block in adrenal mineralocorticoid and glucocorticoid production is present, the steroid precursors are diverted towards the androgen pathway, leading to their overproduction and subsequent virilisation. The aldosterone and cortisol deficiency leads to a state of adrenal insufficiency, causing hyponatraemia, hyperkalaemia, acidosis and circulatory collapse (typically between days 5 and 15).

This case illustrates the severest form of 21-hydroxylase deficiency, the so-called 'salt-wasting' subtype, where there is total lack of the enzyme. Partial enzyme deficiency produces a less severe phenotype ('simple virilising') with adequate aldosterone production, and hence no fluid or electrolyte losses, but still with a strong virilising effect. Non-classic 21-hydroxylase deficiency is more common than classic forms of the disease and produces late-onset and mild clinical symptoms (e.g., premature puberty, tall stature, hirsutism, oligomenorrhoea), usually without gross virilisation at birth.

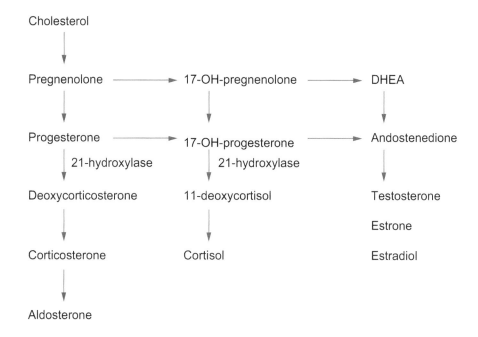

Figure 19.1 Adrenal steroid biosynthetic pathway.

The diagnosis of 21-hydroxylase deficiency can be made with the finding of elevated random 17-hydroxyprogesterone levels in the blood. Measurement of this metabolite after ACTH stimulation can help determine the clinical subtype, with the highest levels seen with salt-wasting forms and lower levels with non-classic deficiency.

Management of this baby involves urgent fluid resuscitation with subsequent glucocorticoid and mineralocorticoid replacement. The other issue is that of the virilised genitalia, which may be surgically corrected in the first year of life.

🔑 KEY POINTS

- Ambiguous genitalia in a newborn may represent either an over-virilised XX female or an under-virilised XY male.
- CAH is usually due to a deficiency of 21-hydroxylase and is a common cause of ambiguous genitalia.
- When 21-hydroxylase is completely deficient, newborns may present with a 'salt-wasting' crisis as a result of their lack of mineralocorticoids.

CASE 20: FATIGUE, WEAKNESS AND WEIGHT GAIN

A 38-year-old woman presents to the general medical clinic complaining of generalised fatigue, muscle aches and pains and disordered menstrual cycles that have been ongoing for the past few months. She has gained around 8 kg in weight in the past year. Her family history is notable for cardiovascular disease in both her parents. The only medications she uses are occasional salbutamol and beclomethasone inhalers for asthma.

Examination

Physical examination reveals an overweight woman (body mass index [BMI] 28). Blood pressure is 146/85. There is evidence of bruising on her arms and abdominal striae. Neurologic examination identifies proximal muscle weakness in the upper and lower limbs.

INVESTIGATIONS

FBC, U+E, LFT	Normal
Random glucose	9.8 mM
Thyroid-stimulating hormone	2 mU/L

QUESTIONS

1. What diagnosis is suggested by the history and examination findings?
2. What investigations are needed to confirm the diagnosis?
3. How may further investigations help delineate between the various causes of this underlying condition?

ANSWERS

In this case, the clinical picture is suggestive of Cushing's syndrome (chronic hypercortisolism). The clinical features of Cushing's syndrome may be categorised by system:

- General (obesity and hypertension)
- Dermatologic (striae, bruising, acne, hirsutism)
- Musculoskeletal (weakness, osteopenia)
- Neuropsychiatric (depression, emotional upheaval)
- Reproductive (menstrual disturbance, reduced libido, impotence)
- Metabolic (glucose intolerance, diabetes, hyperlipidaemia)

Other signs that the physician should look out for include a 'cushingoid' facies ('moon' face), facial plethora and supraclavicular and cervical fat deposits ('buffalo hump').

Appreciation of the hypothalamo-pituitary-adrenal axis allows us to understand the causes of Cushing's syndrome. Corticotrophin-releasing hormone (CRH) is produced in the hypothalamus and stimulates the anterior pituitary to produce adrenocorticotropic hormone (ACTH). The latter acts on the adrenal cortex to produce glucocorticoids (cortisol) and mineralocorticoids (aldosterone). Hence, the causes of Cushing's syndrome are categorised as either ACTH-dependent or ACTH-independent. The most common cause of the former is an ACTH-producing pituitary adenoma (the term Cushing's *disease* is used in this case), while ectopic production of ACTH (e.g., paraneoplastic phenomenon in small cell lung cancer) is another. The most common ACTH-independent cause (and indeed the most common cause overall) is exogenous steroid therapy. Less common ACTH-independent causes include a cortisol-producing adrenal neoplasm and adrenal hyperplasia.

The first stage in the evaluation of suspected Cushing's syndrome is biochemical confirmation of the diagnosis. This is achieved with a low-dose or overnight dexamethasone suppression test (i.e. failure to suppress cortisol levels after a steroid dose), midnight serum or salivary cortisol levels (elevated in Cushing's but low in healthy individuals) or 24-hour urinary free cortisol levels. All three have similar specificities of ~90%, but the specificity is much lower with the latter test (40–50%), compared to nearly 100% for a low-dose dexamethasone suppression test.

Once the diagnosis of Cushing's *syndrome* is made, the priority is to determine its cause. The first step would be to exclude exogenous use of glucocorticoids before moving on to measure plasma ACTH levels (to determine ACTH dependence). In the case of normal ACTH levels, imaging of the adrenal glands by CT or MRI is needed to identify the type of adrenal lesion (e.g., adenoma, carcinoma). With elevated ACTH levels, prompt pituitary imaging via MRI should be performed to look for a pituitary *macro*adenoma. In the presence of a radiologically normal pituitary, CRH stimulation with measurement of ACTH via bilateral inferior petrosal sinus sampling can be used to identify a pituitary *micro*adenoma. Additionally, a high-dose dexamethasone suppression test may help, with suppression of cortisol levels seen in Cushing's disease but not in cases of ectopic ACTH secretion or an adrenal tumour. If a paraneoplastic syndrome is suspected, CT imaging of the chest, abdomen and pelvis will be required to look for a primary tumour.

🔑 KEY POINTS

- Causes of Cushing's syndrome are either ACTH-dependent or ACTH-independent.
- A low-dose dexamethasone suppression test may be used to confirm the diagnosis of Cushing's syndrome.
- Measurement of ACTH levels can help distinguish between the various causes.

CASE 21: HYPERTENSION IN A YOUNG WOMAN

A 42-year-old woman is referred by her GP to the cardiology clinic, as her blood pressure is poorly controlled. She was first diagnosed with hypertension 5 years ago and started angiotensin-converting enzyme (ACE) inhibitor therapy. However, her blood pressure has never been adequately controlled despite addition of a calcium channel blocker. The patient believes the cause to be her stressful job as a lawyer. There is no significant family history, and she denies taking any other medications.

Examination

Vital signs are T 36.8°C, HR 75 and regular, BP 155/85, RR 17, 98% O_2 saturation on room air. Cardiac, respiratory, abdominal and neurologic examinations are unremarkable.

INVESTIGATIONS

FBC, LFT	Normal
Sodium	144
Potassium	3.2
Urea	3.6
Creatinine	80
Thyroid-stimulating hormone	2 mU/L

QUESTIONS

1. The cardiologist thinks there may be a secondary cause to hypertension in this case. What are the causes of secondary hypertension?
2. Given the clinical findings and results of the investigations, which cause is most likely and why?
3. What further tests are required to confirm and establish this diagnosis?

ANSWERS

According to the latest National Institute for Health and Care Excellence (NICE) guidelines, hypertension is defined as blood pressure of 140/90 mmHg or higher that is confirmed by home or ambulatory blood pressure monitoring. In the majority of patients, there is no clear cause ('essential hypertension') but a secondary cause is present in around 5–10% of cases. Secondary hypertension should be considered in young patients, those with very high blood pressure (>180/110 mmHg), absence of risk factors for essential hypertension, a history of hypertensive emergencies and severe or progressive target-organ damage (e.g., deteriorating renal function) and where there are particular symptoms or signs suggestive of an underlying cause (e.g., palpitations, flushing). Here, the fact that our patient was first diagnosed with hypertension in her 30s and that it is still poorly controlled is an indication that a secondary cause should be considered.

The causes of secondary hypertension may be categorised as follows:

- Renal, including renal parenchymal disease, renal artery stenosis and renin-producing tumours
- Endocrine, including primary aldosteronism, Cushing's syndrome, phaeochromocytoma, acromegaly and hypothyroidism or hyperthyroidism
- Cardiac (coarctation of the aorta)
- Neurologic, particularly raised intracranial pressure and stress
- Other, including obstructive sleep apnoea and drugs (e.g., steroids, non-steroidal anti-inflammatory drugs [NSAIDs])

Primary aldosteronism refers to increased production of aldosterone by the adrenal cortex, most commonly caused by an adenoma (Conn's syndrome) and sometimes by bilateral adrenal hyperplasia. This leads to excess retention of sodium, and subsequently water, consequently expanding extracellular fluid volume, and thereby leading to higher blood pressure. Aldosterone is responsible for stimulating potassium excretion; hence the finding of hypokalaemia.

There are three steps in working up a suspected case of primary aldosteronism: (1) screening, (2) diagnosis and (3) elucidating the cause. Screening is performed by measuring the aldosterone:renin ratio, which would be very high (>2000) in hyperaldosteronism as a result of feedback suppression of renin secretion. Subsequently, a confirmatory diagnostic test is needed, such as a fludrocortisone suppression test or a saline infusion test. The principle is that fludrocortisone should suppress aldosterone levels in normal individuals, while in the saline infusion test, sodium loading should inhibit aldosterone secretion. Once primary aldosteronism is confirmed, imaging of the adrenal glands (via CT or, occasionally, MRI) is needed to identify an adenoma or to exclude a functional adrenocortical carcinoma.

🔑 **KEY POINTS**

- The majority of cases of hypertension are idiopathic, but around 5–10% are due to a secondary cause.
- Clues suggesting a secondary cause include young age of onset, very high blood pressure, hypertensive emergencies and specific symptoms (e.g., flushing, palpitations).
- Primary aldosteronism is one cause of secondary hypertension and may be screened for by measuring the aldosterone:renin ratio.

CASE 22: NAUSEA, VOMITING, WEAKNESS AND PARAESTHESIA

A 48-year-old woman presents with a 1-week history of recurrent nausea and vomiting. She reports vomiting up to 12 times a day, aggravated by eating and drinking, and generalised fatigue and muscle weakness "all over". She describes paraesthesia in the distal extremities of her limbs. Her other medical problems include asthma, insulin-dependent diabetes mellitus, hypertension and gastro-oesophageal reflux disease.

Examination

There is reduced skin turgor and dry mucous membranes. There is some epigastric tenderness, but the abdomen is otherwise soft and non-tender, with normal bowel sounds. Digital rectal examination demonstrates good sphincter tone.

INVESTIGATIONS

	Sodium	140
	Potassium	1.9
	Urea	7.5
	Bilirubin	15
	Creatinine	170
	Corrected calcium	2.23
	Phosphate	1.0
	Magnesium	0.55
	Alanine aminotransferase	28
	Alkaline phosphatase	35
	C-reactive protein	42
ABG:		
	pH	7.48
	pO_2	10.8
	pCO_2	5.9
	HCO_3	31
	Base excess	+8

ECG: Rate 98 beats per minute, sinus rhythm, flattened T waves

QUESTIONS

1. How is serum potassium regulated within the body?
2. What are the causes of hypokalaemia?
3. What risks and complications are associated with hypokalaemia?

ANSWERS

The normal serum (extracellular) potassium ranges from 3.5 to 5.5 mM, with intake of around 60 mmol equalling excretion by the cortical collecting duct of the kidneys (50 mmol) and faeces (10 mmol). In the case of chronically impaired kidney function, the body adapts to increase the excretion of potassium in faeces.

There are several causes of hypokalaemia, but fundamentally they result from three processes: (1) reduced K^+ intake, (2) transcellular movement of K^+ and (3) increased K^+ excretion. Movement of potassium from the extracellular to intracellular compartment is seen with an alkalosis (K^+ and H^+ tend to move in opposite directions, so when H^+ moves out of cells to correct an alkalosis, K^+ moves in), insulin treatment, use of β-agonists (hence why salbutamol can be used to treat hyperkalaemia) and in refeeding syndrome. Increased excretion of potassium may occur via the kidneys (e.g., diuretics, diuretic phase of acute renal failure, mineralocorticoid excess), or via extra-renal means (e.g., diarrhoea, vomiting, excess sweating, villous adenomas of the rectum).

This patient's hypokalaemia was most likely a result of vomiting, which caused excess loss of potassium from gut contents. Other contributing factors could include antihypertensives such as loop diuretics (e.g., furosemide), which inhibit potassium reabsorption via the $Na^+/K^+/2Cl^-$ cotransporter in the thick ascending limb of the loop of Henle. The patient was also on insulin and salbutamol, which promote influx of potassium into cells through the Na/K-ATPase channel. The metabolic alkalosis also likely contributed.

Hypokalaemia leads to hyperpolarisation of membranes, resulting in an impaired ability to fire action potentials. This may particularly affect the heart with risk of subsequent arrhythmia. Indeed, ECG changes are observed with hypokalaemia, including ST depression, T wave depression or inversion, prolongation of the PR interval, and a prominent U wave. Other consequences of hypokalaemia include constipation, ileus, rhabdomyolysis and respiratory muscle weakness resulting in ventilatory failure in the most severe cases. With an impaired ability to concentrate urine, patients may also develop a nephrogenic diabetes insipidus, which results in polydipsia and polyuria with dilute 'pale' urine.

The main aim in treating hypokalaemia is to identify and manage the underlying cause (e.g., discontinue offending drugs, alleviate vomiting and diarrhoea). Potassium replacement is frequently required, and generally 140 mmol is needed over 24 hours. It may be given intravenously to start, but regular measurement is required to titrate the level of replacement. High doses of intravenous potassium can irritate peripheral veins and should always be diluted (e.g., in normal saline, which is also required to rehydrate the patient).

🔑 **KEY POINTS**

- Normal serum potassium ranges between 3.5 and 5.5 mM.
- When dealing with potassium, always remember to think of H^+, since the two often go in opposite directions.
- Causes of a low potassium level include reduced intake, transcellular movement of potassium into the intracellular compartment and increased excretion of potassium.
- ECG changes may be seen with hypokalaemia, and there is an increased risk of arrhythmia.

CASE 23: ERECTILE DYSFUNCTION IN A YOUNG MAN

A 36-year-old man presents to his GP complaining of reduced libido and erectile dysfunction that has been ongoing for a few months. He also gives a vague history of headaches increasing in frequency over the past few weeks. He denies weight loss and otherwise does not suffer from any medical problems. He is on no regular medications, apart from occasional ibuprofen for headache.

Examination

Cardiac, respiratory, and abdominal examinations are unremarkable. Testicular size is 10 mL by orchidometry. Neurologic examination is positive for bitemporal hemianopia.

 INVESTIGATIONS

Full blood counts, renal function, electrolytes and liver function are all within normal limits. Further tests are sent with the results pending.

? QUESTIONS

1. What are the causes of hypogonadism in men?
2. What is the likely diagnosis in this case, given the history and examination findings? What investigations should be performed to confirm this?
3. What are the management options for this man's underlying condition?

ANSWERS

The finding of reduced testicular volume (normal testicular volume in post-pubertal men is 15–25 mL) is indicative of hypogonadism, a term that implies defective functional activity of the gonads. Hypogonadism in men can either be primary (i.e. an intrinsic testicular problem) or secondary to an underlying cause. In primary hypogonadism, there is loss of feedback suppression of gonadotrophins (luteinising hormone [LH] and follicle-stimulating hormone [FSH]) owing to low testosterone levels, hence the term *hypergonadotrophic hypogonadism* is used. Causes of primary hypogonadism are either congenital (e.g., Klinefelter's syndrome, testicular agenesis, enzyme defects such as 5-α-reductase deficiency) or acquired (e.g., mumps orchitis, bilateral testicular injury or torsion, irradiation to the testes and effects of cytotoxic drugs). A number of conditions may lead to secondary hypogonadism, including pituitary disorders (tumours and hypopituitarism), hypothalamic disorders (e.g., Kallman's syndrome), obesity and drugs.

Here, the findings of headache and bitemporal hemianopia are strongly suggestive of a pituitary tumour. The visual field defect results from suprasellar extension of the pituitary gland, leading to compression of the optic chiasm, where the nasal fibres from each retina decussate (these carry inputs from the temporal fields of vision). In the context of hypogonadism, reduced libido, and erectile dysfunction, a prolactin-secreting adenoma (prolactinoma) is the most likely diagnosis. Prolactinomas are the most common type of pituitary adenoma, accounting for 60% of cases. Hyperprolactinaemia leads to these symptoms via interference with the secretion of gonadotropin-releasing hormone (GnRH) by the hypothalamus. Testosterone production is downregulated, leading to hypogonadotropic hypogonadism. In women, this may manifest as amenorrhoea or infertility, while gynaecomastia and galactorrhoea may also be seen.

The first step in working up this man should include measurement of serum prolactin. Baseline assessment of thyroid function would be useful, as primary hypothyroidism is a common cause of hyperprolactinaemia. Subsequently, MRI of the brain would be indicated to look for an adenoma. This would help classify the tumour as a microadenoma (<10 mm) or macroadenoma (≥10 mm), though the presence of a visual field defect is indicative of the latter. This categorisation is useful, as it helps govern whether treatment is required (microadenomas do not always need it, whereas macroadenomas generally do).

Treatment of prolactinoma is either medical or surgical. Dopamine agonists, such as bromocriptine or cabergoline, form the mainstay of treating microadenomas and macroadenomas, as they suppress prolactin secretion. Trans-sphenoidal surgical resection is a curative option for microadenomas and as a debulking method for macroadenomas. Reasons for considering surgery include tumour growth despite optimum medical treatment, inability to tolerate dopamine agonists, and persistent optic chiasm compression on optimal medical therapy.

🔑 **KEY POINTS**

- Hypogonadism in men can either be primary (due to an intrinsic testicular problem) or secondary to a condition that interferes with the hypothalamo-pituitary-testicular axis.
- Prolactinomas are the most common form of pituitary adenoma and may present with infertility, reduced libido, and gynaecomastia.
- Management of prolactinoma is usually with dopamine agonists, which inhibit prolactin secretion.

CASE 24: A YOUNG MAN WITH 'HIGH CHOLESTEROL'

A 38-year-old man is advised to see his GP by his new private health insurer, as his baseline blood tests showed that he had "too much cholesterol in his body". He does not suffer from any active medical problems. His father died suddenly at age 53 of an unclear cause, and his two brothers developed type 2 diabetes in their 40s. He is an ex-smoker with a 10 pack-year history.

Examination

General examination reveals an overweight man (body mass index [BMI] 28), with presence of a bilateral corneal arcus. Blood pressure is 135/75. The rest of the examination is unremarkable except for the presence of tendon xanthomas on his hands.

🔍 INVESTIGATIONS

	FBC	Normal
	U+E	Normal
	LFT	Normal
Fasting bloods:		
	Total serum cholesterol	8 mM
	LDL cholesterol	5 mM
	HDL cholesterol	1.5 mM
	Triglyceride	1.2 mM

❓ QUESTIONS

1. Give a brief account of lipid metabolism.
2. What are the causes of hyperlipidaemia? Which cause is the most likely in this case?
3. What is the pathophysiology underlying the most likely cause, and what are suggestive treatment options for this patient?

DOI: 10.1201/9781003242697-25

ANSWERS

The principal lipids in plasma are fatty acids, triglycerides (TGs), and cholesterol. These are transported in plasma in association with proteins, with free fatty acids carried by albumin and other lipids circulating in complexes, termed *lipoproteins*, that have a non-polar lipid core and a surface layer of phospholipids, cholesterol and apolipoproteins. Lipoproteins are classified based on their density, increasing from chylomicrons to very low-density lipoproteins (VLDLs), intermediate-density lipoproteins (IDLs), low-density lipoproteins (LDLs) and high-density lipoproteins (HDLs). As density increases, less TG is present, with increasing amounts of cholesterol and proteins.

Chylomicrons are formed from dietary fat, and their function is to transport TG to the tissues. VLDLs are the primary transport mode for endogenous TG, and as TGs are released to tissues by the action of lipoprotein lipase, they become denser to form IDL and then LDL. LDL carries the majority of plasma cholesterol, which may be taken up by macrophages, a pathogenic event of atherosclerosis. LDL also binds to receptors in the liver, with subsequent lysosomal degradation leading to release of cholesterol intracellularly, which is excreted into bile. The metabolism of HDL is complex, but essentially it mediates 'reverse cholesterol transport' by taking up cholesterol from senescent cells and transferring it to remnant lipoprotein particles that are eventually cleared by the liver.

Hyperlipidaemia is one of the key modifiable risk factors for the development of atherosclerosis. It may either be primary, arising from a genetic disorder, or secondary to other conditions, including hypothyroidism, diabetes mellitus, obesity, nephrotic syndrome, renal and liver failure, drugs (e.g., thiazides, antiretrovirals) and alcohol.

In this case, the man has high levels of total and LDL cholesterol. Given his young age, potential family history, and the clinical findings of tendon xanthomata and corneal arcus, a primary hyperlipidaemia is likely to account for this. The likely diagnosis is familial hypercholesterolaemia (FH), which is an autosomal dominant disorder of LDL metabolism, usually arising from mutations in the LDL receptor leading to reduced uptake by the liver. The homozygous form of the disease is rare and presents in childhood; our patient is more likely to have the heterozygous form, which is reasonably common, with a prevalence of approximately 1 in 500. It typically presents in adulthood with total cholesterol >7.5 and LDL cholesterol >5; a family history of early coronary artery disease or hypercholesterolaemia in a close relative is also required to make the diagnosis. Tendon xanthomas, which are essentially deposits of cholesterol, are pathognomonic.

The management of FH involves lifestyle changes (dietary restriction and regular exercise) and medications, principally using statins, ezetimibe (which inhibits intestinal cholesterol absorption), bile acid sequestrants and the newer PCSK9 inhibitors.

🔑 **KEY POINTS**

- LDL is the principal lipoprotein responsible for transporting cholesterol in the body and is cleared by the liver, with excretion of cholesterol in bile.
- Mutations in the LDL receptor cause FH, which presents with hyperlipidaemia, hypercholesterolaemia, early-onset vascular disease and tendon xanthomas.

CASE 25: RASH AFTER A BONE MARROW TRANSPLANT

A 45-year-old man presents to the haemato-oncology clinic with a rash. He was diagnosed with acute myeloid leukaemia a year ago and received an allogeneic bone marrow transplant for relapsed disease 28 days ago. He also complains of abdominal pain and worsening vomiting and diarrhoea. He is taking cyclosporin.

Examination

The patient has a fever of 38.3°C. There are confluent faint, erythematous, blanching macules with indistinct borders involving the palm and dorsum of both hands, with sparing of the metacarpophalangeal and proximal interphalangeal joints. There are also perifollicular erythematous macules on the upper trunk. There is prominent desquamation, and rubbing the skin results in exfoliation.

General examination reveals scleral icterus. His cardiorespiratory examination is unremarkable. He is tender in the epigastrium and right upper quadrant.

 INVESTIGATIONS

Blood tests are taken, but the results are pending.

? QUESTIONS

1. Based on the clinical findings, suggest a differential diagnosis.
2. Discuss the pathophysiology of the likely diagnosis.
3. What investigations are required?
4. Outline the principles of treatment in this case.

ANSWERS

After a bone marrow transplant (and any associated chemotherapy), the main risks are infection (from low white cell counts and the use of immunosuppressants, such as cyclosporin), bleeding (from low platelet counts) and graft-versus-host disease (GVHD). The causes of a rash in this setting can be a viral, bacterial or drug exanthem; GVHD; or toxic epidermal necrolysis. Given that this patient also has a fever, diarrhoea, vomiting, abdominal pain and signs of jaundice, he may also have an underlying gastroenteritis or liver pathology.

An erythematous rash that develops on the palms or soles of the feet of a patient 10–30 days after a bone marrow transplant is characteristic of GVHD. The pathophysiology of GVHD is still not completely understood, but three requirements for it to occur are proposed:

1. The graft contains immune cells (T cells).
2. The host expresses antigens that are different from those in the donor.
3. The host is unable to mount an immune response to eliminate the donor cells.

Essentially, donor T cells recognise host antigens as foreign or 'non-self' and provoke an immune response also involving B cells and leading to production of inflammatory cytokines such as tumour necrosis factor alpha (TNF-α) and interleukin (IL)-1. As the patient's immune system is designed to be suppressed to allow engraftment of the recipient bone marrow, this response is directed against the patient's own body.

GVHD is a potentially life-threatening problem that can occur in up to 80% of successful allogeneic bone marrow transplants. It may also occur in a milder form in up to 10% of autologous engraftments, where it is hypothesised that chemotherapy exposes self-antigens, which the immune system did not recognise before.

Clinically, GVHD manifests like an autoimmune disease with a macular-papular rash, jaundice, hepatosplenomegaly, and ultimately organ fibrosis. It classically involves the skin, gastrointestinal tract, and the liver. Further investigations in this patient would include a full blood count, measurement of renal function and electrolytes and liver function tests. A skin biopsy would allow histological grading and assessment of the severity of the disease.

Depending on severity, treatment of acute GVHD may involve topical and intravenous steroid therapy, immunosuppression (e.g., cyclosporine), or biologic therapies targeting TNF-α (e.g., infliximab, etanercept), a key inflammatory cytokine. Resolution often takes more than 1 month, and patients should be carefully monitored for opportunistic infections.

Prognosis is related to response to treatment. The mortality of patients who completely respond can still be around 20%, and the mortality in those who do not respond is as high as 75%.

🔑 **KEY POINTS**

- The complications of a bone marrow transplant include infection, bleeding and GVHD.
- Fever and a rash in a patient who recently received chemotherapy or is using an immunosuppressant should be investigated thoroughly and has a broad differential diagnosis.
- GVHD is a type IV, T-cell–mediated hypersensitivity reaction by the graft against the host.
- GVHD is potentially life-threatening and is more common in allogeneic bone marrow transplants.

CASE 26: A FALL ON AN OUTSTRETCHED HAND

A 55-year-old woman presents to the emergency department after slipping on an icy road and falling on her outstretched right hand. She complains of pain in her right wrist that has not responded to simple analgesia and has been unable to use her right hand since falling. She has a history of polymyalgia rheumatica, though has not had a flare-up for a couple of years. She is a non-smoker.

Examination

The patient is haemodynamically stable. She is tender on palpation of the right wrist joint and the ulnar styloid. There is no evidence of any neurovascular compromise.

 INVESTIGATIONS

Plain radiograph of the wrist: transverse fracture of the distal radius with minimal dorsal displacement of the wrist; there is also a fracture of the ulnar styloid.

The fracture is reduced; a back-slab is applied, and the patient is told to return to the fracture clinic in 2 weeks.

? **QUESTIONS**

1. What is the name given to this fracture, and what suspicion should its occurrence raise?
2. What investigations should be arranged in clinic and why?
3. Does the patient require any treatment, and what are the various options in management?

DOI: 10.1201/9781003242697-27

ANSWERS

A fracture of the distal radius with dorsal displacement of the distal fragment describes a Colles fracture, and is classically caused by a fall on the outstretched (extended) hand. The presence of a Colles fracture, especially in a relatively young individual, should raise the question of osteoporosis, since it is one of the three 'fragility fractures' associated with this condition (the other two being a fracture of the neck of the femur and vertebral body fracture).

Osteoporosis is characterised by reduced bone mass and microarchitectural disruption with a resultant reduction in bone strength and predisposition to fracture. It is defined by a reduction in bone density of 2.5 times or greater from the standard deviation of a young adult reference mean (i.e. T score ≤ −2.5). Bone density is governed by the rates of bone formation and breakdown: bone mass accrues through adolescence and reaches a peak in early adulthood, remaining relatively stable until around the fourth decade. Beyond this age, bone mass declines as a result of increased osteoclastic and reduced osteoblastic activity and does so at a faster rate in women as a result of oestrogen deficiency (oestrogen inhibits osteoclasts).

Osteoporosis may therefore be "primary" (post-menopausal in women) or secondary to an underlying condition that accelerates the above process. Secondary causes are:

- Endocrine (e.g., thyrotoxicosis, glucocorticoid excess, hyperparathyroidism)
- Nutritional (e.g., vitamin D deficiency, malabsorptive conditions such as coeliac disease)
- Drugs (principally steroid use)
- Other (e.g., multiple myeloma, osteogenesis imperfecta, rheumatoid arthritis)

In this case, the underlying aetiology may be a combination of chronic steroid treatment for polymyalgia rheumatica and post-menopausal oestrogen deficiency. However, routine investigations to exclude other secondary causes would be worth performing, including a full blood count and ESR (to identify chronic inflammatory conditions such as rheumatoid arthritis), bone profile (for Paget's disease), liver and renal function (vitamin D deficiency in renal failure), thyroid function and a screen for myeloma (Bence Jones proteinuria and serum immunoglobulins). The other important test would be to perform a dual-energy x-ray absorptiometry (DEXA) scan that will be able to measure bone density and confirm the diagnosis.

Treatment of osteoporosis is via a combination of lifestyle and pharmacologic measures. The former includes fall education and prevention, as well as dietary supplementation of calcium and vitamin D. Pharmacologic measures consist of anti-resorptive agents (e.g., bisphosphonates, which inhibit osteoclasts; hormone replacement therapy; and selective oestrogen receptor modulators [SERMs] such as raloxifene) and anabolic agents (e.g., strontium and parathyroid hormone–related peptides such as teriparatide). In this patient, a bisphosphonate would certainly be indicated, given that a fragility fracture has already occurred.

🔑 **KEY POINTS**

- Fragility fractures include fractures of the distal radius (Colles fracture), neck of the femur, and vertebral body.
- Osteoporosis is characterised by a reduction in bone mass and most commonly arises as an age-related phenomenon in women.
- Treatment for osteoporosis usually involves the use of bisphosphonates, which inhibit osteoclastic activity.

CASE 27: A PATIENT IN FOLLOW-UP AFTER A LIVER TRANSPLANT

A 48-year-old gentleman with a history of alcoholic liver disease undergoes an orthotopic liver transplant. The surgery goes well, and the patient has a reasonably uneventful post-operative course. He returns to the transplant clinic 4 weeks later for routine follow-up. He says he has been feeling tired and has not yet returned to work. His wife has noticed that his eyes have turned slightly yellow.

Examination

General examination reveals scleral icterus. Abdominal examination reveals a healed 'Mercedes-Benz' scar in the right upper quadrant. There is no organomegaly or palpable mass.

INVESTIGATIONS	
Haemoglobin	12.0
White cell count	5
Platelets	302
Mean cell volume	105
Bilirubin	48
Alanine aminotransferase	185
Alkaline phosphatase	540
International normalised ratio	1.4

? QUESTIONS

1. What features would indicate that the transplant is being rejected?
2. What are the immunological mechanisms of graft rejection?
3. How can the risk of graft rejection be reduced?

ANSWERS

The leading indication for a liver transplant is alcoholic cirrhosis in adults and biliary atresia in children. To enhance the viability of the graft, transplants of the liver should take place less than 24 hours after the harvest. During this time the organ is kept at 4°C and in a specialised University of Wisconsin preservative solution that facilitates immediate graft perfusion after transplant. The overall 1-year survival of a liver transplant is over 90%, with 10-year survival of around 70%.

Allograft transplant rejection tends to involve the biliary epithelium before the vascular endothelium. Thus, the signs of rejection include increased serum bilirubin (indicating reduced drainage of bile) and deranged liver function tests. If there is suspicion of rejection, other complications of transplantation must be ruled out. These include operative complications (e.g., thrombosis or anastomotic leak) and complications of immunosuppression (infection, especially cytomegalovirus [CMV]) and lymphoproliferative diseases such as Epstein-Barr virus (EBV)–mediated B-cell proliferation. Diagnosis of CMV infection or EBV B-cell proliferation will often require tissue biopsy of the donated organ.

Transplant rejection can be classified by time course, which relates to the underlying immune mechanism:

- *Hyperacute organ rejection* occurs within minutes of the graft perfusion in the operating theatre. It is characterised by a type II antibody-mediated hypersensitivity reaction whereby pre-existing anti-graft antibodies in the recipient bind to foreign antigens. This results in opsonisation with phagocytes engulfing cells that have been marked by antibodies. The antibodies activate complement, which enhances phagocytosis and causes cell lysis. The treatment for hyperacute rejection is immediate removal of the graft.
- *Acute organ rejection* take place a number of weeks after the transplant and is the likely mechanism in this case. It is characterised by cell-mediated toxicity by cytotoxic T cells. This process involves host CD4 T cells recognising foreign antigens (on the graft) and producing cytokines such as interleukin (IL)-2 that stimulate cytotoxic T cells, which are able to initiate apoptosis of the foreign tissue. The treatment for acute rejection includes high-dose steroids.
- *Chronic organ rejection* can take place months to years after the transplant. It is irreversible and characterised by both cell-mediated (cytotoxic T cell) and antibody-mediated (humoral) immune reactions that result in fibrosis and obliteration of the blood vessels of the transplanted organ. As it is irreversible, treatment for chronic rejection is difficult and may include re-transplantation.

All recipients of an organ transplant receive immunosuppressive therapy. This is usually a triple regimen consisting of corticosteroids, azathioprine and cyclosporin or tacrolimus. Triple therapy enables the use of lower doses of each drug, thereby reducing side effects. Corticosteroids downregulate the immune response by inhibiting the principal pro-inflammatory transcription factor, NFκB. Azathioprine is a prodrug that is cleaved into the active metabolite mercaptopurine, which inhibits DNA replication and therefore hinders lymphocyte production and replication. Cyclosporin and tacrolimus (the latter is more potent) both inhibit the protein calcineurin and the production of IL-2 by helper T cells. This results in reduced activation of helper and cytotoxic T cells.

🔑 KEY POINTS

- Allograft transplant rejection involves the biliary epithelium before the vascular endothelium.
- Other complications of transplantation must be ruled out as a differential diagnosis of organ rejection. These include operative complications, infection (especially by CMV), and EBV-mediated B-cell proliferation.
- Hyperacute organ rejection is characterised by a type 2 antibody-mediated hypersensitivity reaction whereby antigraft antibodies in the recipient bind to foreign antigens.
- Acute organ rejection is characterised by cell-mediated toxicity by cytotoxic T cells.
- Chronic organ rejection is irreversible and characterised by both cell-mediated (cytotoxic T cell) and antibody-mediated (humoral) immune reactions.

CASE 28: A MAN WITH POORLY CONTROLLED BLOOD PRESSURE

A 64-year-old man with poorly controlled hypertension for many years presents to his GP with a vague history of generalised weakness, anorexia, bony pains and impotence occurring over the past few months. He has not seen anyone in primary care for the past 5 years. He takes a diuretic for blood pressure control (when he remembers) and has no other medical history.

Examination

Physical examination reveals a thin gentleman (60 kg) with evidence of conjunctival pallor. His blood pressure is 175/95.

🔍 INVESTIGATIONS

Haemoglobin	10.8
White cells	8
Platelets	200
Mean cell volume	90
Sodium	132
Potassium	5.6
Urea	22
Creatinine	375
Alkaline phosphatase	230
Calcium	1.95
Phosphate	1.9

Urine dipstick: +++ protein

Ultrasound of the kidneys: Kidneys measure 8.1 cm and 8.4 cm, respectively, with no obstruction

---

❓ QUESTIONS

1. Given the above results, what can you conclude about this man's underlying condition?
2. What are the common causes, and which is most likely here?
3. Explain all the metabolic abnormalities seen in the blood results. How can the bony pain be explained?

ANSWERS

The most obvious abnormality in the blood tests is a high serum creatinine and urea. Plasma creatinine is the most reliable biochemical test of renal glomerular function and has an inverse relationship with the glomerular filtration rate (GFR). An estimated GFR (eGFR) may be made using the Cockcoft-Gault formula, whereby

$$eGFR\left(mL\:/\:min\right) = \frac{\left(140 - age\right) \times Weight\:in\:kg}{\left[serum\:Cr\right] \times 0.81}$$

An eGFR of 15 mL/min can be calculated for this patient, indicating renal failure. Although we are not given details of the patient's baseline renal function, the renal ultrasound shows small kidneys bilaterally, which suggests that this is long-standing in nature.

Chronic kidney disease (CKD) is characterised by a reduction in GFR over a period of 3 or more months (normal GFR is >90–120 mL/min). It arises from a progressive impairment of renal function with a decrease in the number of functioning nephrons; generally, patients remain asymptomatic until GFR reduces to below 15 mL/min (stage V CKD). Common causes of CKD are (1) diabetes mellitus, (2) hypertension, (3) glomerulonephritis, (4) renovascular disease, (5) chronic obstruction or interstitial nephritis and (6) hereditary or cystic renal disease (e.g., polycystic kidneys). In this case, the most likely underlying cause of the patient's CKD is hypertension.

There are several metabolic consequences of CKD, which give rise to the clinical manifestations illustrated by this case. There is impairment of urinary concentration, leading to polyuria and nocturia. Electrolyte homeostasis becomes deranged as the kidney's primary roles in excreting potassium and H^+ are affected, which can cause hyperkalaemia and acidosis. The kidney's synthetic function in producing erythropoietin (EPO) is reduced, leading to a normocytic anaemia. There is also retention of waste metabolic products, principally urea, and the consequent uraemic state may lead to pericarditis and interference with the hypothalamo-pituitary-gonadal axis (as manifested by impotence in this case). Dyslipidaemia is another complication, and partly explains why cardiovascular disease is the most frequent cause of death amongst patients with CKD.

The bony pains experienced by this patient are also related to renal failure. In CKD, there is phosphate retention with subsequent hypocalcaemia as well, with reduced production of 1,25-dihydroxycholecalciferol (activated vitamin D) by the kidneys. The latter leads to osteomalacia, while the former stimulates increased parathyroid hormone production, leading to secondary hyperparathyroidism. Additionally, in an acidotic state, excess H^+ ions are buffered by bone, causing further demineralisation. These various mechanisms underlie what is termed *renal osteodystrophy*.

The general principles of managing this patient would include close monitoring of renal function, aggressive control of blood pressure, dietary protein restriction and management of cardiac risk factors. Further, as this patient is bordering upon stage V CKD (GFR <15 mL/min), referral to a nephrologist for consideration of renal replacement therapy and/or transplantation would be warranted.

🔑 **KEY POINTS**

- CKD refers to the progressive and irreversible impairment in renal function, leading to a reduction in GFR over at least 3 months.
- The most important causes of CKD include diabetes, hypertension, glomerulone-phritis and renovascular disease.
- Various metabolic abnormalities are seen in CKD, including hyperkalaemia, hyperphosphataemia, hypocalcaemia and a normocytic anaemia.

CASE 29: DIZZINESS ON STANDING UPRIGHT

A 34-year-old woman is referred to the general medical clinic with a 4-month history of increasing fatigue and vague abdominal complaints (including nausea and anorexia). She complains of dizziness on waking up in the morning and has lost 2 kg in weight over this period. She has a history of coeliac disease that is well controlled by a gluten-free diet.

Examination

Vital signs are T 36.4°C, HR 85 and regular, BP 105/70 (sitting) and 95/60 (standing). General examination reveals a thin woman with evidence of pigmentation in the palmar creases, nipples and areolae, as well as around her caesarean scar.

INVESTIGATIONS

Haemoglobin	11.2
White cells	6
Platelets	250
Mean cell volume	85
Sodium	133
Potassium	5.5
Urea	7.0
Creatinine	60
Random glucose	7.2 mM

QUESTIONS

1. Given the above findings, what is the likely diagnosis and why?
2. What test(s) may be used to confirm this diagnosis? Explain their principle(s).
3. Describe some of the aetiologies underlying the likely diagnosis.

DOI: 10.1201/9781003242697-30

ANSWERS

Postural hypotension has several causes, including cardiac and neurologic disease, as well as a drug side effect. In this case, there is absence of a drug history and neurologic or cardiac findings; the most suggestive clinical finding is hyperpigmentation, which is one of the earliest features of primary adrenal insufficiency (Addison's disease). Addison's disease is characterised by the destruction or loss of adrenal cortical function. The adrenal cortex is responsible for producing mineralocorticoids (e.g., aldosterone), glucocorticoids (e.g., cortisol), and adrenal androgens. Normally, cortisol feedback inhibits adrenocorticotropic hormone (ACTH) secretion by the anterior pituitary. ACTH is itself produced from a larger product (pro-opiomelanocortin [POMC]), which is a precursor for melanocyte-stimulating hormone (MSH); hence, when there is cortisol deficiency, the release from feedback suppression causes high levels of ACTH and MSH to be produced, with the latter contributing to hyperpigmentation. Similarly, the deficiency of aldosterone is responsible for postural hypotension (resulting from reduced extracellular fluid volume) and the electrolyte abnormalities seen here (mild hyponatraemia and hyperkalaemia, with a raised urea:creatinine ratio, suggestive of volume depletion).

Various tests may be used to evaluate adrenal insufficiency. Measurement of morning (8 am) serum cortisol can be used to rule out adrenal failure, with a level >550 nM effectively excluding the diagnosis; similarly, a very low level (<50 nM) would point towards adrenal insufficiency. However, in many subjects, these may not be conclusive, and an ACTH stimulation test ('short Synacthen test') is required. In this test, a morning cortisol is measured with administration of synthetic ACTH ('Synacthen') at this time; further cortisol levels are measured at 30 and 60 minutes and should normally exceed 550 nM. Failure to do so, or to at least increase by 200 nM, would indicate adrenal insufficiency. While this test does not tell us whether insufficiency is primary or secondary to pituitary disease, measuring the plasma ACTH level can help determine this—a very high level (>20 pM) would indicate primary adrenal failure due to lack of feedback suppression.

Addison's disease merely signifies the presence of primary adrenal failure, which itself has numerous causes. The most common aetiology is an autoimmune adrenalitis, which, given the history of coeliac disease, is likely in this scenario because of the link with certain human leukocyte antigen (HLA) alleles (DR3/DR4). Other causes of Addison's disease include adrenal haemorrhage (e.g., disseminated intravascular coagulation (DIC) due to *Neisseria meningitidis* infection, the so-called Waterhouse-Friderichsen syndrome), infections (tuberculosis was the most common cause historically), metastatic adrenal disease (especially from a lung primary), and adrenoleukodystrophy (an X-linked disorder afflicting men, characterised by accumulation of very long chain fatty acids in several organs, including the adrenal gland).

🔑 KEY POINTS

- Addison's disease describes primary adrenal insufficiency, which has several causes.
- Autoimmune destruction of the adrenal cortex is the most common cause of Addison's disease and is usually associated with other autoimmune conditions (such as diabetes and coeliac disease).
- A short Synacthen test with concomitant measurement of ACTH levels can be used to diagnose Addison's disease.

CASE 30: SUDDEN-ONSET CHEST PAIN IN A TALL WOMAN

A 32-year-old woman is brought into hospital by ambulance after complaining of severe retrosternal chest pain while on her way to work. Her past history is notable for a spontaneous pneumothorax. She has a 20 pack-year smoking history and takes regular bisoprolol. Her family history is notable for her father dying from a 'heart condition' at age 40.

Examination

General examination reveals a tall, gangly female with a pectus deformity of the chest and ectopia lentis. Abdominal and flank striae are present. HR is 120 and BP 100/60, with RR of 28 and 94% O_2 saturation on 15 L/min. A third heart sound is heard, together with bibasal crackles on auscultation of the chest.

 INVESTIGATIONS

- ECG: ST elevation in leads V1–V6, I and L
- Chest radiograph: widened mediastinum
- Emergency coronary angiography: Dilated aortic root, with a dissection flap and no flow within the left main coronary artery

? **QUESTIONS**

1. How do the angiography findings account for the patient's presentation?
2. In light of the clinical findings, what condition is suspected? Discuss its genetics and pathophysiology.
3. What treatment should the patient receive after this acute episode?

ANSWERS

The clinical presentation here is strongly suggestive of myocardial ischaemia, and the finding of ST elevation in the anterior and lateral leads corroborates this diagnosis. However, the pathology is not purely limited to an acute coronary syndrome, as there are also features of aortic dissection (widened mediastinum and dissection flap on coronary angiography). We may conclude that the dissection flap has closed off the ostia of the left main coronary artery (so this is a type A aortic dissection), thereby leading to cardiac ischaemia. This has also produced likely cardiogenic shock, given the tachycardia and borderline hypotension, the presence of a third heart sound and bibasal crackles.

This constellation of findings is highly consistent with an underlying diagnosis of Marfan's syndrome, a connective tissue disorder inherited in an autosomal dominant fashion with high penetrance but significant phenotypic heterogeneity. Several of the classic features of Marfan's are present, including a pectus deformity of the chest, ectopia lentis, the characteristic body habitus and aortic root dilatation. The positive family history and the history of prior spontaneous pneumothorax support this diagnosis.

The genetic defect underlying most cases of Marfan's is a mutation in the fibrillin-1 gene, which encodes a matrix glycoprotein that forms a key component of the extracellular matrix. Dilatation and weakness of the aortic root arise as a direct result of the loss of vessel elasticity, predisposing individuals to aortic aneurysms and dissection. The inherent weakness in connective tissues provides the explanation for other pathognomonic features of Marfan's, including ectopia lentis (subluxation of the lens), joint hypermobility and chest wall deformity.

The predominant causes of death in patients with Marfan's syndrome are aortic dissection and rupture. All patients should therefore have regular echocardiographic monitoring to chart the rate of increase of aortic diameter, and direct family members should be evaluated for any signs of disease, given the autosomal dominant genetics. Changes in lifestyle designed to avoid sudden or high stresses on the aortic vessel wall are also needed, including the avoidance of intense exertion or exercise. Drugs may also be used to achieve this, with the negative inotropic and chronotropic effects of beta-blockers particularly effective in this regard. Finally, surgery (ideally prophylactic) on the aortic root (a graft repair) has a beneficial effect on survival and is recommended electively in all adults with an aortic root diameter of more than 5 cm.

 KEY POINTS

- Marfan's syndrome is an autosomal dominant disorder caused by mutations in the fibrillin-1 gene, which encodes a matrix glycoprotein in the extracellular matrix.
- The most significant clinical feature of Marfan's syndrome is aortic root dilatation, which predisposes individuals to aortic aneurysms and aortic dissection.

CASE 31: CONCERNS ABOUT THE RISK OF BREAST CANCER

A 33-year-old teacher comes to her GP worried about her risk of developing breast cancer. Both her sisters have recently been diagnosed with the disease at a young age (31 and 38 years), and her mother died of breast cancer at age 45. Additionally, her maternal aunt died of ovarian cancer in her 50s. She does not complain of any breast symptoms at present. Her periods started at age 13, and she has one child who is now 7 years old. She currently takes the combined oral contraceptive pill.

Examination

General and breast examination is unremarkable.

? **QUESTIONS**

1. Given her family history, what is the likelihood that this woman is at increased risk of breast cancer?
2. What are the common forms of hereditary breast cancer that you know? Describe their genetics and how they predispose to oncogenesis.
3. What strategies would you recommend regarding (a) screening for and (b) the prevention of breast cancer in this case?

DOI: 10.1201/9781003242697-32

ANSWERS

Breast cancer is the most common cancer in women in the UK and is the second most common cause of female cancer death. While 15% of women will have at least one close relative (mother, sister or daughter) who is affected by breast cancer, a small proportion of breast cancers (10%) are ascribed as "hereditary breast cancer", owing to germ-line mutations in single, dominantly acting genes. This should be suspected in a family where the following features are present:

- Early-onset breast cancer (<50 years)
- Bilateral cancers
- Particular ethnicity (e.g., Ashkenazi Jews)
- Any male breast cancer
- Other associated cancers (e.g., ovarian, peritoneal or fallopian tube)

The family history here is strongly suggestive of a hereditary predisposition to breast cancer, with three first-degree relatives and one second-degree relative being afflicted by either a breast or related cancer at a young age.

The most common mutations underlying hereditary breast cancer are those in the *BRCA1* and *BRCA2* genes, whose prevalence is estimated at between 1 in 400–800 women. Women harbouring these mutations have a 10- to 30-fold increased risk of breast cancer compared to the general female population. For *BRCA1,* the lifetime breast cancer risk is around 80% with a 40% ovarian cancer risk. There is also a small risk (<5%) of primary peritoneal carcinoma. In the case of *BRCA2,* lifetime risks for breast and ovarian cancer are smaller (40% and 10%, respectively); there is also an increased risk of fallopian tube carcinoma and an excess risk of prostate cancer in men carrying the mutation.

Both *BRCA1* and *BRCA2* encode proteins that have a crucial role in the cell cycle, which helps us understand how mutations accelerate oncogenesis. *BRCA1,* on chromosome 17, encodes a protein that is involved in the DNA damage response; in individuals with a germ-line mutation, the wild-type allele is deleted, leading to impaired checkpoint regulation and allowing mutated and damaged DNA to be replicated. Similarly, *BRCA2,* on chromosome 13, encodes a protein that plays a role in homologous recombination, which is one of the mechanisms by which double-strand breaks of DNA are repaired. A mutation in this gene thereby increases the chances that the cell will replicate damaged or mutated DNA.

The first step in evaluating this woman for a possible hereditary predisposition would be genetic testing of affected family members and herself to confirm the presence of a mutation. If this is confirmed, there are two management options: primary prevention and surveillance. The former includes prophylactic mastectomy and/or oophorectomy or chemoprevention with tamoxifen, while the latter involves regular breast self-examination along with frequent physician examination, together with annual radiographic screening by way of mammography and breast MRI.

🔑 **KEY POINTS**

- Ten per cent of breast cancers are hereditary in nature and should be suspected in families with early age of onset of disease and presence of bilateral tumours.
- The most common genetic causes of a hereditary breast cancer are mutations in *BRCA1* and *BRCA2,* both of which are important in the DNA damage response.

CASE 32: SEIZURE IN A NEONATE

A 5-day-old neonate, born via normal delivery, is seen by his mother to have a "seizure" when she is feeding him. She says that he became limp and his arms flexed before being released. The episode ended within a minute without any medical intervention. Routine prenatal scanning had identified cardiac features consistent with tetralogy of Fallot.

Examination

The neonate is cyanotic, with a soft ejection systolic murmur. The physician notes dysmorphic facies, including microcephaly, low-set ears with abnormal folding and increased distance between the medial epicanthi of the eyes. The eyes are downward slanting.

INVESTIGATIONS

FBC	Normal
U+E	Normal
Alkaline phosphatase	80
Corrected calcium	1.25
Phosphate	1.81
Parathyroid hormone	0.35

QUESTIONS

1. What are some of the causes of a neonatal seizure?
2. Suggest a unifying diagnosis in light of the neonate's medical history, clinical findings and investigation results.
3. Describe the pathology underlying the diagnosis, and explain how it may produce tetralogy of Fallot and this biochemical abnormality.

DOI: 10.1201/9781003242697-33

ANSWERS

Neonatal seizures may be caused by several conditions, the most common of which are hypoxic-ischaemia encephalopathy, intracranial haemorrhage, central nervous system (CNS) infections and metabolic disorders. Seizures may also be benign, typically occurring in the first week of life. Here, blood tests show low calcium, high phosphate and low parathyroid hormone levels, which are suggestive of hypoparathyroidism, and this is the most likely cause of the seizure in this case.

Approximately 40% of serum calcium exists in the active ionised form. However, the majority of calcium is bound to proteins such as albumin. Thus the most common cause of hypocalcaemia is hypoalbuminemia, usually caused by reduced synthesis resulting from liver failure or increased protein losses as a result of nephrotic syndrome. Other causes of hypocalcaemia include autoimmune or congenital hypoparathyroidism, vitamin D deficiency and loop diuretics (not thiazide diuretics, which can cause hypercalcaemia).

Tetralogy of Fallot is a reasonably common congenital cardiac anomaly, characterised by (1) significant ventricular septal defect, (2) pulmonic stenosis, (3) over-riding aorta with respect to the septal defect and (4) subsequent right ventricular hypertrophy. The association of tetralogy of Fallot with neonatal seizures (due to hypoparathyroidism) as well as dysmorphic facies is very suggestive of a congenital cause.

The most likely cause for this combination of problems is DiGeorge syndrome. DiGeorge syndrome is caused by a deletion in chromosome 22q11 (affecting the gene *TBX1*). This results in defects in neural crest cell migration and their derived tissues, notably the third and fourth branchial pouch. Embryologically, the third branchial pouch is responsible for the development of the inferior parathyroid glands and the thymus, whereas the fourth branchial pouch develops into the superior parathyroid glands. Neural crest migration is also critical for the development of the heart, ascending aorta and pulmonary trunk.

Clinically, erroneous development of the parathyroid glands results in hypocalcaemia, which can present as neonatal seizures, tetany, proximal muscle weakness or mental state changes. Hypoplasia of the thymus gland results in T-cell deficiency and recurrent viral or fungal infections. Congenital cardiac anomalies such as tetralogy of Fallot are caused by problems with neural crest cell migration. Of note, DiGeorge syndrome is the second most common cause of congenital cardiac abnormalities after Down's syndrome. Other signs include learning difficulties and dysmorphic facies, as described in the case.

DiGeorge syndrome is usually the result of de novo mutations, with 100% penetrance and variable expression. It may also be inherited in an autosomal dominant fashion.

🔑 **KEY POINTS**

- Neonatal seizures are commonly a result of ischaemia, haemorrhage, and metabolic disturbances, or they may be benign.
- Aberrant development of the third and fourth branchial pouches causes DiGeorge syndrome (deletion in chromosome 22q11).
- This is associated with T-cell deficiency (thymic aplasia) and hypocalcaemia (failure of parathyroid development). It is also the second most common cause of congenital heart defects.

Section 2
HISTOPATHOLOGY

CASE 33: A YOUNG WOMAN WITH ANKLE SWELLING AND SHORTNESS OF BREATH

A 25-year-old woman of Indian origin presents to the emergency department with progressive shortness of breath and ankle oedema over the previous 3 months. There is a history of fever with joint pains during her childhood, which was spent in India. She moved to the UK at age 18. There is no family history of note.

Examination

General examination confirms bilateral, pitting pedal oedema and mild clubbing of the fingers but no cyanosis. Cardiac examination reveals a rumbling mid-diastolic murmur heard best at the apex and a decrescendo early diastolic murmur heard best in end expiration at the left sternal edge. There are fine basal crepitations at both lung bases.

INVESTIGATIONS

ECG shows features consistent with left atrial enlargement. A chest radiograph shows mild cardiomegaly, and an echocardiogram is booked.

QUESTIONS

1. What is the relevance of fever and joint pains in childhood?
2. Why is there a delay in the appearance of the cardiac symptoms?
3. What complications may arise from this condition?

ANSWERS

A history of fever and joint pains in childhood suggests rheumatic fever following group A (beta-haemolytic) streptococcal infection. The immune response to the bacterial antigens cross-reacts with cardiac valvular and connective tissue elements in the joints and other sites. It must be emphasised that cardiac valvular pathology is due to a type II (immune mediated) hypersensitivity reaction and not direct bacterial infection. The characteristic presentation includes migratory polyarthritis of large joints, carditis, subcutaneous nodules, erythema marginatum of the skin and Sydenham's chorea. Blood investigations typically show a raised ESR or the presence of anti-streptolysin O (ASO) antibody.

The most common valve to be involved is the mitral valve, followed by the aortic valve. The murmurs found in this patient reflect this, being indicative of mitral stenosis (mid-diastolic murmur) and aortic regurgitation (early diastolic murmur). The mitral valve is most frequently affected, as it is the valve across which the greatest pressure difference arises. The continued immunologic damage and fibrosis may progress over years to cause deformity of the valves. This is the reason for the late manifestation of symptoms of valvular heart disease, although features of myocarditis may be present in the acute phase of rheumatic fever. Initial valve damage results in mitral prolapse and with time the valvular damage takes the form of thickening of the leaflets and fusion of commissures and of chordae tendinae.

Inflammation of all three layers of the heart is termed pancarditis. If this is caused by rheumatic heart disease, pathognomonic Aschoff bodies may form in all three layers of the heart, but predominantly the myocardium. Aschoff bodies are granulomas with giant cells (mainly macrophages), which can develop into Anitschkow's cells, which represent activated enlarged macrophages.

The signs and symptoms of valvular disease depend on the valves involved and the severity of involvement. Cardiac failure may develop, accompanied by cardiac hypertrophy and dilatation. In a tight mitral stenosis, the left atrium becomes dilated and a mural thrombus may form. Arrhythmias such as atrial fibrillation (which may arise as a result of left atrial enlargement) may lead to thromboembolic complications. Damaged cardiac valves are also susceptible to infective endocarditis, which can worsen the valvular insufficiency and also result in infective emboli to the brain, kidneys, spleen (left-sided lesions) and lungs (right-sided lesions).

 KEY POINTS

- Rheumatic heart disease results from a type II immune-mediated hypersensitivity reaction to group A beta-haemolytic streptococci.
- It most commonly affects the mitral valve, causing prolapse in early stages of the disease and stenosis later on.
- Pathognomonic lesions that affect all three layers of the heart in rheumatic heart disease include Aschoff bodies and Anitschkow's cells, which represent granulomas with giant cells (macrophages).

CASE 34: CHEST PAIN AND SUDDEN DEATH

A 70-year-old man is working in his garden when he suddenly experiences crushing central chest pain, starts sweating profusely and feels short of breath. An ambulance is called, but he collapses in the interim and becomes unresponsive. Cardiopulmonary resuscitation is commenced by the paramedics and continued until they reach hospital, where no output can be restored and the patient is declared dead. The coroner requests that a post-mortem examination be carried out.

Examination

External examination of the body is unremarkable. The heart is of mildly increased weight compared to the normal expected weight (up to 0.5% of body weight). The heart valves are normal, and there is concentric thickening of the left ventricle. The coronary arteries show marked eccentric thickening and calcification of their walls, resulting in such narrowing that only a pinpoint lumen can be seen at one site in the right-sided coronary artery.

? QUESTIONS

1. How is sudden cardiac death defined, and what are the main causes?
2. What is the most likely cause of death in this patient?
3. What are the aetiology and pathogenesis of the likely cause of death?
4. If the patient had been successfully resuscitated, what complications might have occurred?

ANSWERS

Sudden cardiac death is defined as unexpected death from a cardiac cause early after the onset of symptoms, usually within 1 hour. The most common causes of sudden cardiac death include ischaemic heart disease and myocardial infarction or, especially in younger patients, dilated or hypertrophic cardiomyopathy. Other causes include aortic valve stenosis, mitral valve prolapse, myocarditis, pulmonary hypertension, congenital structural abnormalities or, when all of these conditions and other non-cardiac causes of sudden death have been excluded, hereditary or acquired abnormalities of the conduction system. Irrespective of the underlying cause of sudden cardiac death, the common mechanism of death is a lethal arrhythmia triggered by irritability of the myocardium even if the abnormality or injury is distant from the conduction system. These conditions often do not cause symptoms, and sudden death may be the first presentation.

The cause of death in this patient is ischaemic heart disease. This term encompasses related presentations of myocardial ischaemia and includes myocardial infarction, where the degree and duration of interruption of blood supply are sufficient to cause death of the heart muscle, or angina, a lesser form where the heart muscle does not become infarcted. Since myocardial ischaemia of up to 30 minutes may be reversible, features of an acute infarct would not necessarily be seen at autopsy.

Ischaemic heart disease is the most common cause of death in industrialised countries. The dominant cause of ischaemic heart disease is reduced perfusion of coronary arteries relative to myocardial requirement, and in over 90% of cases reduced perfusion is the result of atherosclerosis of the coronary arteries with progressive narrowing of the affected coronary artery. Such atherosclerotic plaques, which commonly show calcification, may rupture ('acute plaque change') and result in overlying thrombosis, which may completely interrupt perfusion, or progressive stenosis of the coronary artery may lead to critical narrowing (usually defined as a pinpoint residual lumen or narrowing of more than 75%).

Myocardial infarction, also known as a 'heart attack', implies death of heart muscle from ischaemia. Whether ischaemia of the heart muscle results in infarction depends on the location and severity of the coronary artery narrowing, the rate at which it develops, the extent of collateral blood supply and the metabolic needs of the heart muscle (this explains why angina or infarction often occurs following exertion).

Great progress has been made in the timely diagnosis and treatment of myocardial infarction, and as a result the overall mortality of myocardial infarction has sharply declined over the last 50 years. In general, patients with previous infarcts, diabetes mellitus or higher age are less likely to survive an infarct, whereas those who do commonly develop one or more complications, some of which may be life threatening in themselves. These include heart failure (which may be early or late), arrhythmias, rupture of the heart muscle with collection of blood in the pericardial sac (cardiac tamponade), pericarditis, extension of the infarct, mural thrombosis and embolism (e.g., a stroke) or valvular dysfunction due to papillary muscle rupture.

🔑 KEY POINTS

- Sudden cardiac death is defined as death occurring within 1 hour of the onset of cardiac symptoms.
- The most common cause of sudden cardiac death in the middle aged and elderly is ischaemic heart disease.
- Patients who survive a myocardial infarct may suffer from complications such as heart failure, arrhythmia and cardiac tamponade, which may all cause death some time after the infarct.

CASE 35: AN ELDERLY MAN WITH SEVERE BACK PAIN

A 77-year-old man phones '999' after experiencing severe backache. The paramedics arrive to find him in severe pain, cold and clammy. While at his house, they note that he smokes and also elicit a history of hypertension. He is tachycardic and hypotensive en route to hospital, and intravenous fluids are started.

Examination

At the emergency department, his observations are HR 120, BP 90/60, RR 26, O_2 92% on room air. The physician is uncertain about the presence of an expansile mass in the abdomen, but examination is hampered by an obese body habitus. Before further imaging or treatment could be commenced, the patient has a cardiac arrest. Cardiopulmonary resuscitation is commenced but proves unsuccessful.

In view of the sudden, unexplained death, the case is referred to the coroner and an autopsy is performed. This shows extensive haematoma in the retroperitoneum.

? QUESTIONS

1. What is the diagnosis?
2. What are the risk factors for this condition?
3. Where else can this condition be seen?

ANSWERS

The autopsy demonstrates massive haemorrhage into the retroperitoneum from a ruptured abdominal aortic aneurysm (AAA). The definition of an aneurysm is an abnormal focal permanent dilatation of all the layers of a blood vessel. An AAA is defined when the aortic diameter, as measured below the level of the renal arteries, is one and a half times normal. Women have smaller aortas, but for convenience, more than 3 cm qualifies as aneurysmal.

The main risk factors for aneurysm formation are male gender, smoking, hypertension, Caucasian/European descent and atherosclerosis. Although atherosclerosis is a risk factor and both diseases share common predisposing factors, there are also differences. Atherosclerosis is primarily a disease of the intima, the innermost layer of the vessel wall, whereas in aneurysms, there is degeneration of the media, the middle layer. The mechanisms are not fully understood, but inflammation, oxidative stress and inappropriate enzyme activation result in degradation of tissue matrix, collagen, and elastin. The weakened wall progressively dilates, and with increasing diameter, the tension in the wall increases, as does the risk of rupture. The annual risk of rupture equals and begins to outstrip the risk of dying from surgery when the aneurysm exceeds 5.5 cm. This is the size above which surgical repair is recommended, comorbidities permitting. A UK national screening programme will eventually (by way of abdominal ultrasound) target all men over the age of 65.

Clinical examination for an expansile, as opposed to a merely pulsatile, mass is helpful, but not always reliable. Ultrasound and computed tomography are the preferred imaging modalities. In some AAAs, incipient rupture may be heralded by a 'sentinel' leak that is contained by haematoma—this can be misdiagnosed as back strain or ureteric colic. Catastrophic rupture, as in this case, presents with hypovolaemic shock and carries a dismal prognosis. The aorta is retroperitoneal, so the pain may be felt in the back, flank and groins as well as the abdomen.

Aneurysmal change can occur in any vessel, including the iliac, femoral, and popliteal arteries, albeit more rarely. More proximally, thoracic aortic aneurysms share a similar pathogenesis, but in the ascending aorta, a different form of degeneration known as cystic medial necrosis is also described. Late-stage syphilis and inherited collagen defects such as Marfan's syndrome are associated with thoracic aneurysms.

Aneurysms of a different pathogenesis can occur in the cerebral circulation, sometimes called berry aneurysms due to their appearance, which, if they rupture, cause subarachnoid haemorrhage. Coronary artery aneurysms occur in Kawasaki's disease, a form of autoimmune vasculitis. The term aneurysm is also used to refer to the thinning and dilatation of the heart wall following myocardial infarction.

The term 'false aneurysm' is used to refer to contained collections of blood immediately outside a vessel but where there is still a direct communication through a defect in the vessel wall. This usually occurs following trauma, commonly iatrogenic trauma caused during arterial puncture required for percutaneous transarterial interventional procedures.

🔑 **KEY POINTS**

- An aneurysm is an abnormal focal permanent dilatation of all the layers of a blood vessel.
- Some of the risk factors for aneurysm formation are male gender, smoking, hypertension and atherosclerosis.
- Rupture of a previously unsuspected aortic aneurysm is a life-threatening condition.

CASE 36: INCREASED BREATHLESSNESS AND SUDDEN DEATH

His wife finds her 68-year-old husband dead in his bed. During the last year of his life he had slept on a bed in the downstairs living room, as he was unable to walk upstairs due to extreme and worsening breathlessness. As his death is sudden and somewhat unexpected, the general practitioner discusses the case with the local coroner, who decides that a post-mortem examination is required.

Examination

At autopsy the most significant feature on external examination is that of an abnormally shaped chest with an increase in the anteroposterior diameter and mild peripheral oedema. The most significant abnormality on examination of the organs is seen in the lungs, which are voluminous and meet in the anterior mediastinum, where they overlap the heart anteriorly. There are also large air-filled and intact bullae seen in subpleural positions and more strikingly at the apex. There is also mild thickening of the right ventricular heart muscle.

? QUESTIONS

1. What is the most likely cause of death?
2. Describe the aetiology and pathogenesis of this condition.
3. How may this condition lead to death?

ANSWERS

The most likely cause of death is respiratory failure resulting from chronic obstructive pulmonary (or airway) disease (COPD). COPD refers to two separate disorders, chronic bronchitis and emphysema, which commonly co-exist and are characterised by progressive and irreversible damage to the lungs and airways that limits airflow to and from the lungs. Cigarette smoking is, by far, the most common causative factor of COPD. COPD is a major cause of morbidity and ranks within the ten most common causes of death worldwide. Although there are typical clinical and radiological features of COPD, this diagnosis, in life, is made on the basis of lung function tests (spirometry).

Emphysema is the result of chronic inflammation of the airways and lungs, with release of inflammatory mediators resulting in destruction of alveolar walls. As a result of this the alveolar surface area needed for gas exchange is reduced and there is loss of structural support for intrapulmonary airways, which are then more likely to collapse and trap air within the lungs. This chronic over-inflation of the lungs leads to the classic barrel-shaped enlargement of the chest (increased anteroposterior diameter). Typical clinical features of emphysema include progressive dyspnoea (usually a relatively late sign), coughing, wheezing and weight loss. Patients typically show prolonged expiration due to entrapment of air, tend to sit hunched forwards, and breathe through pursed lips.

Depending on the predominant distribution of tissue damage, emphysema is classified as centriacinar, panacinar, paraseptal or irregular. In general, centriacinar emphysema is the result of cigarette smoking, with reactive oxygen free radicals from cigarette smoke causing inactivation of antiproteases. The resultant functional antiprotease deficiency is responsible for tissue damage.

A further cause of emphysema, more commonly with a panacinar distribution, is α-1 antitrypsin deficiency, a genetic abnormality in which homozygous patients have a congenital deficiency in α-1 antitrypsin and are therefore unable to counteract the destructive effects of inflammatory mediators on lung tissue. These patients develop emphysema at an earlier age and may also develop chronic liver disease.

Chronic bronchitis is the result of chronic irritation of the airways caused by inhaled particles in cigarette smoke or, less commonly, dust from substances like grain and cotton. Chronic bronchitis presents with hypersecretion of mucus in the airways, a persistent cough, and frequent infective exacerbations. Recurrent infections are a secondary rather than causative feature of chronic bronchitis but an important factor in the chronic nature of the illness.

Emphysema and long-standing severe chronic bronchitis may lead to respiratory failure or cause pulmonary hypertension, with the latter leading to increased strain on the right ventricle. This culminates in cor pulmonale (pure right-sided heart failure). Both conditions can result in sudden death. Rupture of a bulla can result in pneumothorax, which may also result in sudden death, especially in a patient with already compromised respiratory function.

🔑 **KEY POINTS**

- COPD encompasses emphysema and chronic bronchitis and is most commonly caused by cigarette smoking.
- The predominant abnormality in emphysema is destruction of alveolar walls, whereas chronic bronchitis is characterised by chronic inflammation of the airways.
- Complications of COPD include respiratory failure, cor pulmonale with right-sided heart failure, or pneumothorax, all of which may result in sudden death.

CASE 37: A WORSENING COUGH AND HAEMOPTYSIS

A 54-year-old male who is a long-term smoker presents with a history of worsening cough with haemoptysis. He confesses to a poor appetite and weight loss of 5 kg over the past 3 months. He works as a builder and is unable to say whether he may have been exposed to asbestos.

Examination

The patient appears emaciated. There is conjunctival pallor and digital clubbing. Examination of the chest reveals reduced breath sounds and a stony dull percussion is noted in the left lower zone. There is no palpable lymphadenopathy or abdominal organomegaly.

INVESTIGATIONS

- Hb 11.6, MCV 85, WCC 6.7, PLT 240, Na 135, K 3.8, Ur 4.5, Cr 80, Corr Ca 2.75, Bili 4, AST 20, ALT 15, ALP 85.
- Chest radiograph: Moderate left pleural effusion with a bulky left hilum.

QUESTIONS

1. What is the most likely diagnosis in this case?
2. What is the importance of the raised serum calcium?
3. What investigative techniques may be employed in confirming the diagnosis?

ANSWERS

This presentation is very typical of lung cancer. The patient is a smoker presenting with worsening cough and haemoptysis, and while these features may be seen in non-neoplastic lung disease such as chronic obstructive pulmonary disease (COPD) and tuberculosis (TB), the rapid progression of symptoms is more likely to be associated with malignancy. The findings on the chest radiograph further strengthen the diagnosis. Loss of appetite and weight loss with associated anaemia are indicative of a wasting process, although not specifically lung cancer.

The hypercalcaemia observed in this patient likely represents a paraneoplastic syndrome, which results from ectopic hormone secretion by the tumour. Squamous cell carcinomas in particular are associated with producing PTH-related proteins, which are responsible for the hypercalcaemia. Other paraneoplastic syndromes seen with lung cancer include Lambert-Eaton myasthenic syndrome, which causes muscle weakness as a result of autoantibodies against calcium channels in neuromuscular junctions. Peripheral neuropathy and acanthosis nigricans may also be manifestations of lung carcinoma. Apical lung lesions (Pancoast tumours) may invade the cervical sympathetic chain and produce Horner's syndrome with enophthalmos, ptosis, miosis and anhidrosis.

The diagnosis of lung carcinoma may be made on clinical and radiological findings, but confirmation by examination of tumour tissue or cells is essential. This is because the treatment and prognosis are strongly linked to the histological type of lung carcinoma. Tumour tissue may be obtained in the following ways:

1. Bronchoscopic biopsy of the lung mass.
2. Bronchoscopic brushing of the lung mass and/or saline washing (lavage) of the bronchi and lung for deep-seated tumours. These may be done in combination with biopsy to increase the chances of obtaining diagnostic material or as an alternative to biopsy if the tumour is very vascular and therefore likely to bleed excessively.
3. In patients with mediastinal lymphadenopathy, endobronchial ultrasound combined with transbronchial needle aspiration (EBUS TBNA) provides not only the tissue diagnosis but also establishes the lymph nodal stage of the carcinoma. In addition, the cells obtained from this procedure may be used for analysis of molecular markers such as EGFR, KRAS, RET, ALK and ROS1, which predict the responsiveness of lung adenocarcinoma to certain groups of chemotherapeutic agents. This allows the selection of the most appropriate therapy for individual patients (targeted therapy).

    Next-generation sequencing (NGS) may be performed to cover not only the previous markers but also a number of other genes with the possibility of discovering future targets.

    Patients who are negative for chemotherapeutic targets may be tested for PD-L1 status and considered for immunotherapy.
4. Cells may also be obtained from the pleural fluid for diagnosis, staging and molecular testing.

The most common histological types of lung cancers are squamous cell carcinoma, adenocarcinoma and small cell carcinoma (SCLC). These may be present in variable proportions within the same tumour. Squamous cell carcinoma and adenocarcinoma are sometimes referred to as non–small cell lung carcinoma (NSCLC) to distinguish them from SCLC, which is a form of neuroendocrine carcinoma and is responsive to a different group of chemotherapeutic agents.

The strong association between smoking and lung carcinoma (SCLC and squamous cell carcinoma) is well proven. Adenocarcinoma is seen to arise in the vicinity of scars in the lung secondary to infarcts and inflammatory conditions. Whilst surgery may be effective for squamous cell carcinoma and adenocarcinoma, chemoradiotherapy is the treatment of choice for SCLC.

🔑 KEY POINTS

- Lung carcinoma is a common form of carcinoma, which should be readily suspected on its clinical and radiological features.
- Advances in bronchoscopic techniques in obtaining tumour tissue have made accurate diagnosis and staging easier.
- Histological typing and molecular analysis of the tumour are central to tailoring the appropriate therapy for individual patients (personalised medicine).

CASE 38: A YOUNG MAN WITH SHORTNESS OF BREATH AND HAEMOPTYSIS

A 22-year-old man is brought into the emergency department complaining of a 1-week history of shortness of breath and one episode of haemoptysis. He does not report a fever or any gastrointestinal symptoms. There is no family or medication history of note.

Examination

The patient is tachypnoeic (RR 28) with a blood pressure of 110/70 mmHg. He is afebrile, and there is no cyanosis or jaundice. A further episode of haemoptysis is observed during assessment.

 INVESTIGATIONS

- Urine dipstick: 3+ blood
- Urine cytology: Tubular epithelial casts
- Chest radiograph: Multiple bilateral lung shadows
- Bloods: Ur 13.5, Cr 175

? QUESTIONS

1. What are the likely causes of this clinical presentation?
2. What is the best test to confirm the diagnosis?
3. What is the treatment for the underlying condition?

ANSWERS

The patient's clinical presentation may be caused by an infection involving the lungs with systemic spread. In the absence of fever or signs of infection, other possibilities should be considered, but blood and urine cultures should always be performed to exclude sepsis. The presence of tubular epithelial urinary casts is indicative of renal parenchymal damage, and in conjunction with the respiratory symptoms and radiographic findings, the possibility of Goodpasture's syndrome should be considered.

Goodpasture's syndrome is an immunologically mediated disorder (type 2 hypersensitivity) which affects the lungs and kidney. Antibodies are directed against native tissue antigens of the glomerular basement membrane (GBM) and lung alveolar septa, accounting for the renal and pulmonary manifestations seen in the condition. It usually presents in young adults and teenagers and may be triggered by a viral infection or exposure to chemicals (e.g., dry-cleaning solvents). Smoking has been implicated as a co-factor, and there is a genetic association with the HL-DR2 subtype.

While testing for anti-GMB antibodies is required in the workup for suspected Goodpasture's syndrome, the best investigation to confirm the diagnosis is a renal biopsy. This would be expected to show focal proliferative glomerulonephritis in early cases and crescentic glomerulonephritis in rapidly progressive cases. Linear deposits of immunoglobulins (IgG) and complement (C3) would be seen along the GBM in the kidney and also in alveolar septa in the lungs. The GBM antigen responsible is a component of the non-collagenous domain (NC1) of the alpha-3 chain of collagen type 4.

There are other conditions that damage the glomerulus due to an intrinsic tissue antigen (Heymann's nephritis) and those due to planted antigens (drugs, infections). In Heymann's nephritis, the pattern of deposition of immune complexes in the glomerulus is granular and interrupted rather than the linear pattern seen with Goodpasture's syndrome.

The treatment for this condition is plasmapheresis, which clears anti-GBM antibodies and other chemical mediators circulating in the blood. Immunosuppressive therapy limits further antibody production and prevents lung and renal bleeding. Some patients may require dialysis or renal transplant if the kidney damage is severe. Goodpasture's syndrome was a rapidly fatal disease in the 1970s, but prompt diagnosis and treatment have changed the prognosis in recent years.

 KEY POINTS

- Goodpasture's syndrome involves a type 2 hypersensitivity reaction that results in a combination of renal and pulmonary manifestations.
- The anti-GBM antibody results in rapid damage to the renal GBM and the lung alveolar septa.
- Treatment involves plasmapheresis and immunosuppression, without which the disease may be fatal.

CASE 39: SUDDEN-ONSET WEAKNESS AND DYSPHASIA

A 70-year-old man with a history of type 2 diabetes mellitus, hypertension and hypercholes-terolaemia is brought into hospital with sudden onset of expressive dysphasia and right arm and leg weakness.

Examination

On examination, the patient has right hemiparesis with reduced power Medical Research Council (MRC 3/5) in the right arm and right leg.

INVESTIGATIONS

An urgent computed tomography (CT) scan of the brain is arranged. The images are reviewed, and an intravenous drug treatment is administered. Within an hour, there is partial resolution of the symptoms.

QUESTIONS

1. What is the diagnosis?
2. What treatment is most likely to have been given, and why was the urgent CT scan required?
3. What risk factors are associated with this condition?
4. What blood vessel and what territory of the brain was involved?

ANSWERS

The likely diagnosis in this case is an ischaemic stroke. Stroke refers to an acquired focal neurological deficit caused by an acute vascular event. The neurological deficit persists beyond 24 hours, in contrast to a transient ischaemic attack (TIA), where symptoms resolve before 24 hours, although the distinction is now blurred with the advent of thrombolysis. The term cerebrovascular accident is sometimes used synonymously with stroke, but many dislike the connotations of inevitability it implies, in conflict with the treatable nature of the predisposing factors and, to an extent, the acute event itself.

Strokes are broadly categorised into ischaemic and haemorrhagic types, with the majority being ischaemic. The pathophysiology in a haemorrhagic stroke is rupture of a blood vessel causing extravasation of blood into the brain substance with tissue damage and disruption of neuronal connections. The resulting haematoma also compresses surrounding normal tissue.

In most ischaemic strokes, there is thromboembolic occlusion of vessels due to underlying atherosclerosis of the aortic arch and carotid arteries. In 15–20% of cases, there is atherosclerotic disease of smaller intrinsic blood vessels within the brain, most commonly the lenticulostriate arteries, occlusion of which results in so-called lacunar infarcts. A further 15–20% are due to emboli from the heart.

Although ostensibly an anastomosing ring connecting the main blood vessels of the brain, the circle of Willis has limited capacity to provide collateral blood supply in the event of sudden occlusion of one branch. At certain levels of ischaemia, neurons cease to function but remain viable and can recover with restoration of blood flow, which is the situation in a TIA. The area at the periphery of an infarct (penumbra) is therefore potentially salvageable with thrombolysis. In this case, thrombolytic therapy by means of tissue plasminogen activator (t-PA) was given to the patient. A CT scan was required to exclude conditions such as haemorrhagic stroke or brain tumours, which are contraindications to thrombolysis.

If the critical ischaemic threshold is crossed, irreversible neuronal damage occurs. Dead neurons release destructive cellular enzymes and excitatory neurotransmitters into the extracellular fluid, damaging neighbouring neurons and inciting the release of inflammatory mediators from the surrounding microglia and astrocytes. Infarction and liquefactive necrosis ensue.

Where atherosclerosis is the main underlying pathological process, other non-modifiable risk factors include age, gender, race, and genetic factors. In contrast, modifiable risk factors for atherosclerosis include hypertension, diabetes mellitus, hyperlipidaemia and smoking. For embolic disease, atrial fibrillation, heart failure and endocarditis are known risk factors.

The blood supply to the brain can be divided into an anterior circulation, supplied by the anterior and middle cerebral arteries (branches of the internal carotid artery), and a posterior circulation, consisting of the posterior cerebral arteries, which is fed by the vertebrobasilar arteries. The territory and the extent of the infarct influence the prognosis; here, expressive dysphasia and right hemiparesis are attributable to infarcts in Broca's area and the motor cortex, both frontal lobe territories supplied by left middle cerebral artery.

KEY POINTS

- Stroke refers to focal neurological deficit arising from an acute vascular event, which may be either ischaemic or haemorrhagic.
- Early thrombolysis has revolutionised the clinical management of stroke.
- The neurological deficit corresponds to the blood vessel involved and the territory of the brain that it supplies so that accurate localisation of the lesion is possible.

CASE 40: NUMBNESS, WEAKNESS AND CLUMSINESS

A 35-year-old female presents to her general practitioner with increasing clumsiness and weakness in both legs, developing over a period of several weeks.

Examination

On examination, the GP notes mild stiffness and hyperreflexia and refers her to a neurologist for further investigation.

When questioned in more detail by the neurologist, the patient recalls previous episodes of paraesthesia in her arms a few years previously, as well as a separate incident of unilateral visual field loss associated with eye pain. She did not seek medical attention on either occasion, as the paraesthesia was only a mild nuisance, and she attributed the visual symptoms to irritation from her contact lens.

 INVESTIGATIONS

MRI brain: Lesions with high T2 signal intensity in the periventricular region.

? **QUESTIONS**

1. What is the likely diagnosis?
2. What is the most common pattern of this disease?

ANSWERS

The likely diagnosis is multiple sclerosis (MS). MS is an immune-mediated demyelinating disorder, the aetiology of which is unclear. Several weak genetic factors, mainly in the genes regulating inflammatory mediators, are thought to interact with environmental factors. The idea of environmental influences was supported by observation that the incidence of MS was greater at higher latitudes, with the place of childhood up to the age of 15 being key. Influences such as vitamin D and various viruses have been implicated, but none of these have been proven conclusively.

The name of the disease derives from the multiple inflammatory lesions seen histopathologically that eventually progress to sclerosis. These are typically located in the periventricular areas and mainly, but not exclusively, affect white matter (myelin is macroscopically white). However, the cerebellum, spinal cord, and optic nerve can be affected too. Inflammation and destruction of the myelin results in degeneration of the nerves associated with the myelin covering. Neurological deficit occurs because neurons fail in the same way that chewing the insulation of a fine wire causes failure of ability of the wire to transmit electrical signals.

Diagnosis, however, is rarely made on biopsy and is primarily based on clinical features with radiological corroboration. The lesions and plaques enhance with MRI contrast (gadolinium-based compounds). Cerebrospinal fluid protein electrophoresis may show oligoclonal immunoglobulin G bands, a manifestation of the inflammation, but as lumbar puncture is an invasive procedure, this investigation is increasingly reserved for cases where MRI is contraindicated or where there is diagnostic doubt.

Classically, MS is described as having lesions separated in space and clinical attacks separated in time. These symptoms are myriad and include visual problems (optic neuritis), as well as sensory, and motor symptoms include bladder, bowel, and sexual dysfunction. The most common clinical pattern is the relapsing-remitting form, where there are episodes of neurologic deficit with recovery or near resolution in between. The majority of patients with this form develop progressive disease, usually after 10–15 years.

Other patterns include primary progressive MS (10% of cases). This pattern responds poorly to immunosuppressive and immunomodulatory treatments, where most therapeutic efforts have been concentrated. The progressive-relapsing form accounts for 5% of cases, which resembles primary progressive MS but shows fluctuations superimposed on a progressive course.

 KEY POINTS

- MS typically presents as a remitting and relapsing neurological disorder.
- The multifocal damage and partial regeneration of the myelin sheath of neurons underlie the pathology of this condition.
- Clinical diagnosis is supported by radiological appearances of typical periventricular lesions and also examination of the cerebrospinal fluid, which demonstrates oligoclonal IgG protein bands.

CASE 41: FORGETFULNESS AND DISORIENTATION

A 75-year-old man is referred to the care of the elderly outpatient clinic with progressive changes in mood and behaviour occurring over the past few months. His wife has noticed that he has become increasingly disorientated and forgetful, and is sometimes unable to recall things such as the names of various members of his family. He has a history of bowel cancer and is currently in remission.

Examination
Neurological examination shows preservation of sensory and motor functions but reduced cognitive functions. Mini-Mental State Examination (MMSE) is 19 out of 30.

 INVESTIGATIONS

A CT scan is ordered and shows evidence of cortical atrophy but no significant cerebral vessel disease.

? QUESTIONS

1. What is the clinical diagnosis based on these data?
2. Why are the clinical features not localised to well-defined areas of the brain?

DOI: 10.1201/9781003242697-43

ANSWERS

The features described above are most suggestive of Alzheimer's disease. This is character-ised by progressive deterioration of cognitive functions (dementia), which is beyond what is expected as part of normal ageing. Alzheimer's disease is the most common dementia in all age groups, but is usually seen over the age of 65 years. It can only be diagnosed when other causes of cognitive decline are ruled out. Other causes of dementia include Pick's disease, vascular dementia, diffuse Lewy body disease, Creutzfeldt-Jacob disease and neurosyphilis.

Examination of the brain tissue is diagnostic, but clinical and radiological features allow accurate diagnosis in the vast majority of cases. For instance, Pick's disease is characterised by an earlier age of presentation (40–60 years) and mainly with behavioural and speech defects. It is associated with excessive deposition of one or two isoforms of tau proteins within ballooned cells (Pick cells) in the brain, typically in the frontal and parietal lobes. In contrast, Alzheimer's is characterised by a later age of presentation, mainly with memory loss and, histologically, by deposition of all six isoforms of tau proteins extensively across the brain.

Signs and symptoms of vascular dementia typically present following a stroke and then show a 'stepped' pattern of progression. Single photon emission computed tomography (SPECT) and positron emission tomography (PET) provide evidence of metabolic activity of the brain and help in distinguishing vascular dementia from Alzheimer's.

Lewy body disease overlaps between Alzheimer's and Parkinson's diseases due to loss of cho-linergic and dopaminergic neurons, respectively. Visual hallucinations and rapid eye move-ment (REM) sleep disorders are common. SPECT and PET are helpful investigations in making a clinical diagnosis. Histologically, Lewy bodies are characterised by deposition of alpha-synuclein throughout the brain.

Macroscopic examination of the brain in Alzheimer's disease at autopsy shows a variable degree of cortical atrophy with widening of sulci most pronounced in the frontal, temporal, and parietal lobes. There is secondary dilatation of the ventricles due to loss of parenchyma. The main abnormalities include the presence of neurofibrillary tangles, neuritic plaques and amyloid angiopathy. These may be present in smaller degrees in normal elderly people.

The neurofibrillary tangles represent the end stage of a number of degenerative processes and are seen in other neurodegenerative disorders. The neuritic plaques are found in the superficial portions of the cerebral cortex, basal ganglia, and cerebellar cortex and may be centred on blood vessels or clusters of neurons. Amyloid deposition is seen commonly in Alzheimer's disease and is composed of the same amyloid as that in the neuritic plaques. Granulovacuolar degeneration occurs in abun-dance in the hippocampus and olfactory bulb. Hirano bodies are found along the hippocampal pyramidal cells. The widespread distribution of the pathology explains the overall deterioration, rather than symptoms referable to a well-defined area of the brain, as seen with vascular disease.

🔑 **KEY POINTS**

- Alzheimer's disease is characterised by progressive deterioration of cognitive functions (dementia), which is beyond what is expected as part of normal ageing.
- Other causes of dementia include vascular dementia, Lewy body disease, and Pick's disease, which are distinguished by a constellation of signs and symptoms and backed up by investigations such as SPECT and PET.
- Characteristic pathological findings in Alzheimer's disease include atrophy of brain sulci and widening of gyri and, histologically, the presence of neurofibrillary tangles, amyloid deposition and granulovacuolar degeneration.

CASE 42: COFFEE-GROUND VOMITING

A 45-year-old man presents to his GP complaining of a several week history of intermittent epigastric gnawing pain, partially relieved by over-the-counter antacids. There is no history of other medical illnesses or medications. The pain appears to be worsening and has been associated with two days of nausea and vomiting. He describes the contents of his vomit as resembling coffee grounds. The patient also mentions that his stools have become darker and tarrier.

Examination
Abdominal examination reveals a soft abdomen with mild epigastric tenderness, but no masses or organomegaly.

INVESTIGATIONS

An urgent upper GI endoscopy is arranged at the hospital.

QUESTIONS

1. What is the likely diagnosis?
2. What aetiological factors are associated with this?
3. What complications may occur with this condition?

ANSWERS

The likely diagnosis is a bleeding peptic ulcer with resultant haematemesis and melaena. The term peptic ulcer disease covers duodenal and gastric ulcer disease. Classically, gastric ulcers are worse during meals, as eating stimulates acid production, whereas duodenal ulcers are worse after meals, but, in practice, history is unreliable in distinguishing the two.

The aetiologic factors underlying this condition can be thought of as those that increase acid secretion and those that weaken the mucosal barrier. Acid hypersecretion can be caused by hormone-secreting rarities such as systemic mastocytosis, which secrete histamine, or gastrinomas, which secrete gastrin. The latter, when located in the pancreas and associated with peptic ulceration, is known as Zollinger-Ellison syndrome.

One should think of the gastric mucosa as a dynamic system, which responds to injury and possesses the ability to repair itself, rather than as a passive barrier. Many of these functions are mediated by autacoids, in particular prostaglandin E2. Glucocorticoids and non-steroidal anti-inflammatory drugs (NSAIDs) both interfere with production of these protective prostaglandins, with NSAIDs responsible for 20–25% of peptic ulcers. Compromised mucosal defences are also causative in 'stress' ulcers seen in trauma, burns, and other severe illnesses. Smoking and alcohol are recognised 'soft' risk factors.

By far the strongest aetiologic factor is *Helicobacter pylori*, a bacillus that survives the harshly acidic stomach environment by producing urease. This enzyme splits urea into carbon dioxide and ammonia, the latter of which neutralises stomach acid. It also expresses membrane proteins that mediate adhesion to gastric epithelial cells and other proteins that aid evasion of the human immune response.

Asymptomatic carriage of *H. pylori* is present in more than half of the general population. However, only 15–20% of infected individuals develop symptomatic disease. *H. pylori* causes acid hypersecretion and disruption of the gastric mucosa via cytotoxin production and the inflammatory response it elicits. The resulting gastritis manifests as acute inflammation (histologically, neutrophils would be present) along with varying degrees of tissue damage.

Over a long period, chronic blood loss from erosive gastritis may result in anaemia. In contrast, larger ulcers may present as overt bleeding, as in this case. Upper gastrointestinal (GI) endoscopy in this scenario is diagnostic and potentially therapeutic. Gastric biopsy may be taken to determine *H. pylori* status using a rapid urease test—if positive, *H. pylori* should be eradicated with a suitable combination of antibiotics and a proton pump inhibitor (e.g., amoxicillin, clarithromycin, and omeprazole). Anatomically, bleeding ulcers are typically more posterior, whereas ulcers on the anterior surface ulcerate into the peritoneal cavity resulting in perforation and peritonitis.

If *H. pylori* persists, acute gastritis evolves into chronic gastritis with accompanying atrophy of the gastric epithelium and intestinal metaplasia. Bacterial cytotoxins and oxidative stress from ongoing inflammation increase the susceptibility of the gastric epithelium to dysplasia and, ultimately, adenocarcinoma, a recognised long-term complication that has led to *H. pylori* being classified as a carcinogen.

🔑 KEY POINTS

- Peptic ulcers occur when there is either increased acid secretion or when there is weakening of the mucosal barrier.
- The aetiological agent for peptic ulceration is a bacterium, *H. pylori*, and treatment involves antibiotics to eradicate the infection.
- Long-standing chronic gastritis may be associated with atrophy, metaplasia and development of malignancy.

CASE 43: EPISODIC RIGHT UPPER QUADRANT ABDOMINAL PAIN

A 58-year-old female with treated hypertension as her only other medical history presents to her general practitioner with constant right upper quadrant pain and nausea after a particularly rich celebratory meal. She describes previous similar episodes after meals, but she attributed these to indigestion from over-eating. On questioning, she has not noticed skin or conjunctival discoloration. The appearance of her urine and faeces is normal.

Examination
Abdominal examination is unremarkable.

 INVESTIGATIONS

FBC, U+E, LF T: Normal

? **QUESTIONS**

1. What is the likely cause of her symptoms?
2. What factors are associated with this condition?
3. What complications are associated with this condition?

ANSWERS

The clinical history is typical of biliary colic, a common presentation of gallstones. Biliary colic is usually experienced as epigastric (the gallbladder is a foregut structure) or right upper quadrant pain, occurring shortly after protein- or fat-rich meals that stimulate gallbladder emptying. The term colic is a misnomer, as the pain is often constant, caused by mechanical impaction or distension of the gallbladder by gallstones. The explanation is that the gallbladder does not contract in peristaltic waves, or put another way, each wave is several hours apart. Nausea and vomiting may accompany the pain.

Bile is 80–85% water and 10% bile salts, with the remainder made up of mucus, pigments, inorganic salts, lipids, and cholesterol. Bile is supersaturated with cholesterol, which is kept in solution by the bile salts. Gallstones form when there is an imbalance in the constituents of bile or bile stasis. Eighty per cent of stones are mixed cholesterol/pigment stones, about 15% pure cholesterol stones and the remainder pigment stones.

The stereotypical profile of a gallstone patient is summed up by the 4Fs: female, fat, fertile and 40. However, while gallstones are twice as common in females, increasing age is a more important risk factor. Above the age of 60, 10–20% of the Western population have gallstones. Conditions that favour gallstone formation include haemolytic disorders such as sickle cell disease; pregnancy, parenteral nutrition (which abolishes regular emptying), rapid weight loss (which changes the relative proportions of cholesterol and pigment in bile) and loss of bile salts due to terminal ileitis or ileal resection.

Most people with cholelithiasis are asymptomatic, but there is a 1–4% annual risk of developing symptoms or complications. Repeated episodes of biliary colic can result in inflammation of the gallbladder, sometimes with bacterial infection. Such flare-ups are referred to as acute cholecystitis, usually suggested by the presence of fever, systemic malaise, raised inflammatory markers, and peritoneal irritation. The latter is elicited by testing for Murphy's sign, where a hand is placed on the right subcostal area and the patient is asked to inspire. As the diaphragm descends, the liver and gallbladder impinge on the fingers of the examining hand. Murphy's sign is positive if there is sudden cessation of the inspiratory effort due to pain.

Complications depend on the size of the stones. Smaller stones may escape into the common bile duct, but may lodge at the narrowing of the hepatopancreatic sphincter (sphincter of Oddi), obstructing the common bile duct and pancreatic duct and leading to obstructive jaundice and pancreatitis, respectively. Obstructive jaundice can also occur when a larger stone within the gallbladder compresses the common bile duct indirectly, a condition known as Mirizzi's syndrome. Other rare complications include erosion of gallstones into the duodenum or stomach, effectively causing a fistula and gallstone 'ileus', where the escaped gallstone obstructs the small bowel distally.

Once symptomatic, the definitive treatment of gallstone disease is generally surgical via a cholecystectomy.

🔑 **KEY POINTS**

- Biliary colic is caused by mechanical impaction or distension of the gallbladder by gallstones.
- Repeated episodes of biliary colic can result in inflammation of the gallbladder, sometimes with bacterial infection (acute cholecystitis).
- Treatment of persistent symptoms is cholecystectomy.

CASE 44: CHRONIC DIARRHOEA AND FLATULENCE

A 25-year-old Irish woman is referred by her general practitioner to the gastroenterology clinic with a 3-month history of diarrhoea, accompanied by flatulence and weight loss. She reports that her bowels open up to three times each day. She does not report any other symptoms, and there is no history of foreign travel. She has a family history of Graves' disease in her brother.

Examination

Physical examination reveals a thin young woman with evidence of mild conjunctival pallor. Abdominal examination is unremarkable.

 INVESTIGATIONS

Baseline blood tests show a mild microcytic anaemia but nothing else of note. Serological tests are requested, and a biopsy is planned.

? QUESTIONS

1. What serological investigations and biopsy are likely to be requested?
2. What is the underlying disorder, and how is it managed?
3. What long-term risks are associated with this condition?

ANSWERS

The clinical presentation of diarrhoea, flatulence and weight loss is fairly typical of coeliac disease.

Coeliac disease results from sensitivity to gluten, the protein component (gliadin) of grains such as wheat, oat, barley and rye. There is a strong association of coeliac disease with certain human leukocyte antigen (HLA) haplotypes. Deaminated gluten peptides bind strongly to HLA-DQ2 and DQ8, presenting an HLA-gluten peptide complex that activates CD4+ T cells, which produce inflammatory cytokines, including interferon gamma, which leads to flattening of the intestinal mucosa. Indeed, association with these various HLA haplotypes is also seen with other autoimmune conditions, such as type 1 diabetes and autoimmune thyroid disease. The positive autoimmune family history in this case therefore provides a clue to the coeliac diagnosis.

The diagnosis of coeliac disease can be made in the following ways. Firstly, the presence of autoantibodies, namely anti-endomysial or anti–tissue-transglutaminase (TTG) antibodies, favour the presence of coeliac disease. The gold standard, however, is a small intestinal biopsy, typically of the duodenum or jejunum. This would be expected to show atrophy and blunting of villi, accompanied by intraepithelial lymphocytosis. The changes are more marked in the proximal small intestine, as it is exposed to the highest concentration of gluten; hence this is the preferred site for biopsy.

The small intestine is the site of absorption of various nutrients, and hence, coeliac disease can lead to malabsorption of these, leading to various deficiencies. Iron, vitamin B_{12}, and folate deficiencies may produce an anaemia, whilst calcium malabsorption leads to osteomalacia. Lack of fat absorption causes steatorrhea, and also interferes with the absorption of fat-soluble vitamins (A, D, E and K).

Clinical management includes withdrawal of gluten from the diet and demonstration of a subsequent improvement in symptoms and histological findings. Indeed, this would prove the diagnosis. Management of the various features of malabsorption (e.g., iron, vitamin, and folic acid deficiencies) may also be required.

With regard to the complications of coeliac disease, there is a small increase in the long-term risk of malignancies such as intestinal lymphomas (enteropathy-associated T-cell lymphoma [EATCL]) and gastrointestinal and breast carcinomas as well.

 KEY POINTS

- Coeliac disease is caused by sensitivity to the gliadin component of gluten resulting in villous atrophy and blunting in the small intestine.
- The gold standard for diagnosis is jejunal biopsy. Anti-endomysial and anti-TTG are highly specific.
- Treatment involves lifelong abstinence from gluten, including barley (including beer), oats, flour, wheat and rye.

CASE 45: A YOUNG MAN WITH BLOODY DIARRHOEA

A 22-year-old Caucasian male presents to his general practitioner with bloody diarrhoea and mucus on and off over the last few weeks. He does not report a fever or any history of recent foreign travel. On direct questioning, he denies any extra-intestinal symptoms.

Examination

General and abdominal examination is unremarkable. Digital rectal examination is also unremarkable.

INVESTIGATIONS

Baseline blood tests ordered by the GP show a mild normocytic anaemia. The patient is referred for a fast-track colonoscopy, which shows moderate inflammation in the rectum and sigmoid, but the proximal large bowel appears normal. A biopsy series is taken from the rectum to terminal ileum. A stool sample is also sent for culture.

QUESTIONS

1. What is the clinical diagnosis based on the above data?
2. Why is it important to enquire about extra-intestinal symptoms in this patient?
3. What are distinguishing pathological features of this condition?
4. What are the long-term complications?

ANSWERS

Bloody diarrhoea may be caused by acute infections (viral, bacterial or protozoal). Non-infectious causes of haemorrhage into the large bowel include inflammatory bowel disease, ischaemic bowel disease, diverticular disease, polyps, angiodysplasia, haemorrhoids or a bleeding diathesis. The presentation of bloody diarrhoea intermittently over a period of weeks and without any features of infection is suggestive of inflammatory bowel disease (IBD). Left-sided disease on colonoscopy with a sharp demarcation between inflamed and proximally normal mucosa supports this and favours ulcerative colitis.

A history of extra-intestinal symptoms is important because ulcerative colitis and Crohn's disease, the other variant of IBD, may be associated with migrating polyarthritis, ankylosing spondylitis and sacroiliitis. Hepatic involvement by pericholangitis and primary sclerosing cholangitis is seen more commonly in ulcerative colitis. Uveitis and renal obstruction due to retroperitoneal fibrosis may also accompany IBD. Fat and vitamin malabsorption may ensue with Crohn's disease due to involvement of the terminal ileum, as this is where these nutrients are absorbed. IBD is an immunological disorder and with established genetic associations which are, however, different for the two clinical subtypes.

Ulcerative colitis involves the mucosa and submucosa of the rectum, and the inflammation spreads proximally but is typically confined to the colon with occasional backwash ileitis. No normal intervening areas remain. With regeneration of the mucosa, pseudopolypoid appearance develops. A diffuse chronic inflammatory infiltrate is present in the submucosa, and crypt abscesses form as neutrophilic infiltration progresses. There is distortion of the crypt architecture with mucosal ulceration and fibrosis.

Crohn's disease is characterised by transmural inflammation of segments of the gastrointestinal (GI) tract (from the mouth to anus), accompanied by non-necrotising granulomata and fissuring of the mucosa. The intervening segments of the GI tract are normal (skip lesions). Early mucosal lesions (aphthous ulcers) coalesce to produce linear fissures in between surviving mucosa with a cobblestone appearance. The fissures may extend deeply into the bowel producing adhesions or even fistulae.

Crohn's disease may be associated with perforation and strictures, whilst ulcerative colitis may progress to involvement of deeper layers (muscularis propria and neural plexus) with resultant toxic megacolon and potential perforation. However, it is the development of dysplasia and invasive malignancy that poses a long-term risk, more so in patients with ulcerative colitis.

It is assumed that long-standing chronic inflammation is responsible for this increased risk. This is supported by the fact that colon cancer risk increases with longer duration of colitis, the extent of colitis, the concomitant presence of other inflammatory manifestations such as primary sclerosing cholangitis, and the fact that certain drugs used to treat inflammation, such as 5-aminosalicylates and steroids, may prevent the development of colorectal cancer.

The major carcinogenic pathways that lead to colorectal cancer (e.g., chromosomal instability, microsatellite instability and hypermethylation) are seen in inflamed colonic mucosa. Oxidative stress also plays a role, as reactive oxygen and nitrogen species produced by inflammatory cells can interact with key genes involved in carcinogenic pathways such as p53 and the DNA mismatch repair gene.

The risk of carcinoma is 20–30 times higher in patients with pancolitis of more than 10 years' duration compared to the normal population.

🔑 KEY POINTS

- Bloody diarrhoea may be caused by infectious agents (viral, bacterial and proto-zoal) as well as non-infectious conditions (e.g., IBD).
- Ulcerative colitis and Crohn's disease are the two clinical types of IBD.
- Long-standing and extensive IBD is associated with an increased risk of dysplasia and carcinoma of the colon.

CASE 46: ABDOMINAL DISCOMFORT AND GENERALISED WEAKNESS

A 58-year-old man presents to his general practitioner with a 4-week history of generalised weakness and malaise. He also complains of mild abdominal discomfort but cannot identify any change in his bowel habit (he opens his bowels once a day) nor any blood in his stools. There is no family history of note.

Examination

General examination reveals conjunctival pallor. His weight has reduced by 5 kg since it was previously recorded on his last attendance 2 months ago. Abdominal examination is unremarkable. Digital rectal examination identifies soft stool, but no masses.

 INVESTIGATIONS

Baseline blood tests show a mildly microcytic anaemia (Hb 11.5, MCV 78) but no other abnormalities. As a faecal occult blood test is positive, the GP refers the patient for further investigations, which identify a polypoid mass in the caecum, and a biopsy is taken. The remaining large bowel appears normal.

? QUESTIONS

1. What is the likely nature of the polypoid mass and why?
2. What other findings may come to light at colonoscopy?
3. How do right-sided colonic tumours differ in their presentation from left-sided ones?
4. What factors determine the prognosis of patients with colon carcinoma?

ANSWERS

The clinical history and examination point to a progressively worsening condition over a period of a few weeks, which in the absence of features of chronic infection, are suggestive of malignancy.

Occult blood in the faeces and anaemia are due to chronic blood loss from the polypoid tumour, which tends to have a friable surface and bleeds easily. The biopsy will confirm whether the polyp shows epithelial dysplasia only or invasion into the deeper layers of the bowel wall. Histologically, polypoid tumours may be adenomas with dysplasia, which may be low grade or high grade. The term adenocarcinoma is used when invasion is seen into the stalk of the polyp or deeper into the bowel wall. Adenomas may show a tubular, villous or a combination of architecture. The larger the adenoma and the more villous its architecture, the higher is the risk of adenocarcinoma.

Colonoscopy may detect synchronous tumours in other parts of the bowel or identify underlying conditions such as inflammatory bowel disease. Bowel cancer may arise in familial syndromes such as polyposis coli in which the bowel is carpeted with polyps and in which the risk of progressing to invasive malignancy is almost 100%. Long-standing inflammatory bowel disease may also give rise to epithelial dysplasia and progression to malignancy. Inflammatory bowel disease may be variably symptomatic, but there is usually a suggestive clinical history.

Right-sided tumours such as those in the caecum may grow into large polypoid masses due to its large capacity. Those arising in the left-sided colon may give rise to fresh bleeding, mucus in stools, and rectal pain and therefore are more likely to present early.

The prognostic features in colon cancer include the grade or differentiation of the carcinoma, as well as the pathological TNM stage, which includes the depth of invasion (T) and assessment of metastasis to lymph nodes (N) and other organs (M). Grade 1 corresponds to well-differentiated carcinoma and Grade 3 to poorly differentiated. The higher the grade, the worse the prognosis. The pathological stage can be fully assessed only after definitive surgery. Both of these factors are addressed in the modified Dukes' staging of colorectal carcinoma. The presence of lymphovascular invasion and distant metastases are other important prognostic features.

The biopsy in this case demonstrated Grade 3 adenocarcinoma with invasion into the muscle layer of the bowel wall; hence, right hemicolectomy with lymphadenectomy would be the treatment of choice.

KEY POINTS

- Anaemia associated with weight loss and positive faecal occult blood are highly suggestive of bowel cancer.
- Right-sided tumours often present just with anaemia, whereas left-sided cancers are more symptomatic.
- A worse prognosis is rendered by higher-grade tumours (containing less differentiated cells), lymph node involvement and distant metastasis.

CASE 47: ABDOMINAL PAIN IN A PUBLICAN

A 49-year-old pub owner presents to the emergency department with a progressive 2-week history of epigastric pain, nausea, and vomiting. He has no other past medical history, in particular, no previous history of peptic ulcer disease or gallstone disease. On direct questioning, he admits to drinking up to half a 750 mL bottle of spirits a day, i.e. up to 105 units per week (one alcohol unit is 10 mL of alcohol, and the strengths of alcoholic beverages are stated as alcohol by volume or ABV; most spirits are about 40% ABV).

Examination

General examination reveals an overweight gentleman with an identifiable whiff of alcohol. Abdominal examination shows epigastric tenderness, but no peritonism or guarding.

 INVESTIGATIONS

Blood tests show:

- Bilirubin: 28 μmol/L
- Alanine aminotransferase (ALT): 60 IU/L
- Alkaline phosphatase (ALP): 150 IU/L
- Gamma glutamyl transferase: 142 IU/L
- Amylase: 592 IU/L

? QUESTIONS

1. What is the diagnosis?
2. What other differential diagnoses should be considered?
3. What is the most likely cause?
4. What other causes are associated with this diagnosis?

ANSWERS

This is alcohol-induced acute pancreatitis. Taking the history alone, differential diagnoses to be considered include causes of foregut pain such as gastritis, peptic ulcer disease and, given the deranged liver enzymes, gallstone disease and hepatitis.

Pancreatitis is typically diagnosed with a suitable history and a serum amylase of at least three times the upper limit of normal (a mild hyperamylasaemia may be seen in various intra-abdominal pathologies). Lower levels may be consistent with a diagnosis of pancreatitis, as levels decline after 2–3 days. The level of amylase does not correlate with severity of pancreatitis. Lipase is equally valid for diagnosis.

In most series, alcohol and gallstones both account for 30–35% of cases. In the in-patient setting, pancreatitis occurs in about 10% of patients undergoing endoscopic retrograde cholangiopancreatography (ERCP). A significant number of cases, as many as 10–20%, remain idiopathic, although this may reflect the diminishing returns of exhaustive investigation once alcohol and gallstones have been excluded. The remaining 1–2% are caused by hypercalcaemia, hyperlipidaemia, various drugs and toxins, trauma, hypothermia, mumps and autoimmune disease.

In the normal pancreas, self-digestion is prevented by several mechanisms: the enzymes are stored as pro-enzymes, requiring activation by trypsin, itself a digestive enzyme. In addition, the intracellular pH and calcium concentration keep the enzymes inactive. Alcohol and several of the other causes disrupt these mechanisms, resulting in premature activation and leakage of enzymes into the parenchyma. In gallstone disease, small stones or biliary sludge block the ampulla, preventing drainage of pancreatic secretions and forcing pancreatic secretions into the parenchyma.

Regardless of the initiating cause, there is inappropriate activation of enzymes within the parenchyma that creates a cascade of further activation of more unreleased enzymes. The damage caused can be extensive, as the pancreas is a soft, fleshy organ (pan = all, creas = flesh). The inevitable acute inflammation is usually mild and self-limiting, but in about 10% of cases, it is sufficient to result in widespread systemic inflammation and cause compromise of various organ systems. Circulatory collapse, renal failure and adult respiratory distress syndrome may ensue. These severe cases of pancreatitis carry a mortality of up to 10% and should be identified early through a combination of clinical assessment, imaging, and predictive physiological scores (e.g., the modified Glasgow score), so they can be given the best supportive care.

Repeated episodes may result in chronic inflammation with destruction of the pancreas with irreversible morphological changes. The early changes are mainly on a histological level (atrophy and fibrosis), but in later stages are detectable radiologically as calcification. Ultimately, there is both endocrine and exocrine impairment, such that these patients require insulin and enzyme supplementation with meals. With little residual exocrine pancreas remaining, serum amylase is rarely raised in chronic pancreatitis.

🔑 **KEY POINTS**

- Pancreatitis can be diagnosed with severe epigastric pain and a markedly elevated serum amylase or lipase.
- The most common causes of pancreatitis are excessive alcohol intake and gallstones.
- Activation of digestive pancreatic enzymes within the pancreatic parenchyma leads to acute inflammation; chronic inflammation results in irreversible atrophy and fibrosis.
- Remember that pancreatitis displays a broad clinical spectrum from mild disease to pancreatic necrosis that results in multi-organ failure and death. Never underestimate diseases of the pancreas.

CASE 48: ABDOMINAL DISTENSION, LOSS OF APPETITE AND MALAISE

A 56-year-old man presents to his general practitioner with a 2-month history of abdominal distension together with loss of appetite and generalised malaise. He also says that he noticed a few drops of fresh blood in his stool last week. He has a past history of asthma and type 2 diabetes mellitus. He is currently unemployed, and there is no family history of note.

Examination

General examination reveals an undernourished male with mild jaundice and ascites. Abdominal examination identifies prominent blood vessels over the umbilicus and splenomegaly, but the liver is not palpable.

🔍 INVESTIGATIONS

Baseline blood tests show:

Serum bilirubin	51
Alanine aminotransferase	60
Aspartate aminotransferase	100
Serum protein	40

An ascitic tap is arranged and shows that the fluid is a transudate, with no malignant cells being seen on cytological examination.

❓ QUESTIONS

1. What important piece of information has the patient not provided?
2. Is the clinical condition reversible?
3. What other investigations should be performed to ascertain the diagnosis, and how do the findings correlate with the clinical progress of the condition?

ANSWERS

The clinical presentation is one of advanced liver damage. The presence of ascites and jaundice in the absence of features of malignancy suggest alcoholic liver disease (ALD) as the likely cause. A history of alcohol excess often has to be elicited through direct questioning, as the patient will not always be forthcoming with this information.

ALD is associated with fatty infiltration into hepatocytes initially in a centrilobular location. The liver is enlarged, tender, and palpable per abdomen at this stage. These fatty changes are reversible in the early stages of disease if alcohol use is discontinued.

The next step of the disease process is alcoholic hepatitis. This is characterised biochemically by an AST:ALT ratio of more than 1.5 and pathologically by necrotic hepatocytes and cytoplasmic accumulation of cytoskeletal material (Mallory bodies). Some fibrosis commences around the sinusoids and venules.

With continued alcohol-related damage, cirrhosis develops, which is irreversible. Cirrhosis may be defined as organ-wide fibrosis with intervening regenerating nodules of liver tissue. Pathologically this is characterised by a shrunken, misshapen, sclerosed liver that contains micronodules that makes the surface rough. This shrinkage means that the liver may no longer be palpable. Accompanied clinical findings include portal hypertension as a result of regenerating hepatic nodules distorting blood flow in the hepatic parenchyma. This manifests as ascites and opening of collateral blood vessels by portal-systemic blood flow. Manifestations of the latter include prominent veins around the umbilicus (caput medusae), oesophageal varices and life-threatening haematemesis and haemorrhoids with bleeding per rectum. Liver damage also interferes with synthesis of blood clotting factors, which may result in a bleeding diathesis.

Once the ascites has been reduced by paracentesis, a liver biopsy may be performed to confirm the diagnosis of cirrhosis. It would also exclude other contributory metabolic disorders such as Wilson's disease and haemochromatosis.

The fibrosis of blood vessels in the portal and intestinal circulation in the liver results in portal hypertension. The raised haemodynamic pressure within this circulation leads to the outflow of a transudate into the peritoneal cavity. It is also promoted by hypoalbuminaemia, filtration of lymph into the peritoneal cavity and sodium and water retention (secondary hyperaldosteronism). Long-standing portal congestion can lead to splenomegaly.

Metabolic disturbances such as hyperammonaemia result in abnormal neurotransmission in the central nervous system and neuromuscular systems (encephalopathy). This is usually seen in advanced stages of hepatic failure. Hepatorenal syndrome may also develop and is associated with signs of renal failure that typically reverse with improvement in liver function. Long-term survivors of cirrhosis face an increased risk of hepatocellular carcinoma.

KEY POINTS

- ALD and alcoholic hepatitis are reversible processes that involve centrilobular fatty infiltration.
- Continued alcohol abuse results in irreversible cirrhosis, which is characterised by fibrosis and a shrunken liver.
- Portal hypertension causes ascites due to outflow of transudate into the peritoneal cavity. Portosystemic anastomoses may subsequently form, leading to bleeding oesophageal varices and haemorrhoids.

CASE 49: BACK PAIN AND FEVER IN A DIABETIC

A 58-year-old woman presents to the accident and emergency department with a 3-day history of increasing back pain and fevers. The patient is a type 2 diabetic on oral hypoglycaemic agents and suffers from mild hypertension. There is no history of burning micturition or colicky abdominal pain. There is no history of chronic analgesic ingestion.

Examination
The patient is febrile (37.9°C) and appears unwell. There is tenderness over the left loin. There is no anterior abdominal tenderness.

🔍 INVESTIGATIONS

Examination of the urine shows the presence of leucocytic and granular casts. Urine culture is requested. Haematological investigations reveal a mild normocytic normochromic anaemia. Serum creatinine and urea are normal.

An ultrasound of the abdomen is requested and shows atrophic, cystic kidneys with dilated pelvicalyceal systems. The gallbladder, liver and spleen are normal.

❓ QUESTIONS

1. What is the likely cause of the patient's symptoms?
2. What is the significance of casts on examination of the urinary sediment?
3. How do the ultrasound findings reflect the underlying pathology?

DOI: 10.1201/9781003242697-51

ANSWERS

These features are most likely due to an episode of acute pyelonephritis. The patient is diabetic and therefore is predisposed to urinary tract infection, and the symptoms point to an upper tract rather than lower urinary tract infection.

The presence of casts indicates renal parenchymal pathology. Casts may be of different types, and leucocytic casts are indicative of an infective renal parenchymal episode. Renal tubular casts are associated with some types of glomerulonephritis such as systemic lupus erythematosus (SLE), while red blood cell casts are seen in acute renal failure. Granular casts are seen in advanced forms of renal parenchymal pathology (i.e. chronic pyelonephritis). The co-existence of acute symptoms on a background of chronic disease (non-insulin-dependent diabetes mellitus [NIDDM]) suggests acute and chronic pyelonephritis.

The ultrasound appearances closely reflect the underlying pathology. Chronic pyelonephritis is accompanied by damage to the renal parenchyma with resulting atrophy and scarring. Obstruction perpetuates the renal damage, predisposes to infection, and results in dilatation of the pelvicalyceal systems proximal to the obstruction.

Chronic pyelonephritis may be associated with obstruction to the lower tract (posterior urethral valves) or with ureteric calculi. It may also be due to reflux nephropathy, particularly in children. The kidneys are typically coarsely scarred, and if bilateral, the involvement is asymmetric. In chronic glomerulonephritis, on the other hand, renal scarring is symmetric. The coarse scarring in pyelonephritis leaves the calyces blunted and dilated, most marked at the poles where reflux is most pronounced.

Histologically, the tubules would show atrophy and dilatation and their lumina would be filled with eosinophilic casts, imparting a thyroid-like appearance to the renal parenchyma. Loss of tubular concentrating function gives rise to polyuria and nocturia. There is chronic inflammation in the interstitium. In the presence of acute infection, leucocyte casts may be seen in the tubules. Long-standing chronic pyelonephritis may be associated with hypertension due to hyaline arteriosclerosis of the renal interstitial blood vessels. Changes attributable to diabetes may also be seen if this was a predisposing condition. Patients with chronic pyelonephritis and reflux nephropathy may also show focal segmental glomerulosclerosis.

Acute episodes of infection complicate chronic pyelonephritis with the appearance of fever and systemic symptoms. If uncontrolled, this may result in septicaemia and shock, especially in the presence of diabetes or unrelieved obstruction. Hence, prompt recognition and clinical management of the condition are essential.

KEY POINTS

- Acute pyelonephritis is characterised by fever and loin pain, and individuals with compromised immunity are predisposed to this condition.
- Urine examination, including microbiological culture, is helpful in making the diagnosis.
- Chronic pyelonephritis has a very characteristic appearance of asymmetrically contracted, coarsely scarred kidneys.

CASE 50: URINARY PROBLEMS IN AN ELDERLY MAN

A 70-year-old man presents to his general practitioner for a check-up. On direct questioning he admits to increasingly frequent urination, also at night, and difficulty starting to urinate. He denies any pain at urination and has not noticed blood in his urine. He has no significant previous medical history.

Examination and Investigations

The GP requests a blood test for prostate specific antigen (PSA) and performs a digital rectal examination (DRE), which reveals firmness in one lobe of the prostate. The PSA result is received days later and is increased at 8 ng/mL. The patient is referred to a urology clinic, where transrectal prostate biopsies are performed and sent for histological examination.

? QUESTIONS

1. What are the features on biopsy that would suggest a prostate cancer, and how may these changes be graded?
2. Discuss the aetiologic factors underlying prostate cancer.
3. What are the treatment options if this gentleman was found to have prostate cancer?

ANSWERS

PSA is a product of prostatic epithelium and as such is specific to the prostate, which allows a PSA level to be used as a screening test for unsuspected prostate cancer in asymptomatic men. Many laboratories consider a level of 4 ng/mL to be the upper limit of normal, but practice varies. As there is considerable overlap in PSA levels associated with cancer and benign conditions, and because neither DRE nor most imaging modalities used to visualise the prostate (transrectal ultrasound or MRI) are sensitive or specific enough, transrectal or transperineal core biopsies of the prostate are required to confirm the diagnosis.

Microscopic examination of the prostate biopsies in this man showed prostatic carcinoma. The volume (length or percentage of tumour per biopsy) and degree of tumour differentiation are also determined microscopically. Gleason patterns are graded from 1 to 5, with patterns 1 and 2 rarely encountered. Pattern 3 is the most common (well differentiated), followed by pattern 4 (moderately differentiated) and pattern 5 (poorly differentiated). The Gleason score is the sum of the two most prevalent and/or most aggressive growth patterns seen in the tumour. Cancer diagnosed on needle biopsies typically is assigned a Gleason score between 6 (least aggressive) and 10 (most aggressive). For example, a tumour showing a predominant pattern 3 and some pattern 4 would be recorded as Gleason score $3 + 4 = 7$. A tumour with a predominant pattern 3 and some patterns 4 and 5 would be recorded as Gleason score $3 + 5 = 8$ to include the worst area of the tumour in the score.

Prostate cancer is the most common cancer of men and is typically slow growing, with many men remaining asymptomatic and eventually dying of unrelated conditions. A minority of prostate cancers are aggressive and may spread to bone, especially the lumbar vertebrae, or lymph nodes. The aetiology of prostate cancer is not well understood, but several risk factors such as increased age, family history and diet are suspected. Prostate cancer is androgen-dependent, and anti-androgen agents or even oestrogens may be used for treating advanced prostate cancer.

Management options for prostate cancer include active surveillance, surgery, radiotherapy or hormonal therapy. Cancer that is considered to be low risk (low Gleason score, low volume, and confined to the prostate) can in many cases be safely managed through active surveillance. This typically consists of annual PSA tests and future re-biopsy or earlier re-biopsy if the PSA level increases rapidly.

Surgery is usually recommended to those men where the expected benefit of prostatectomy outweighs the risk of side effects such as erectile dysfunction and urinary incontinence. Modern surgical techniques have limited the extent of such adverse effects, and in younger men with higher-risk cancer (larger volume or high Gleason score) that is confined to the prostate, prostatectomy tends to be the best option. Radiotherapy or hormonal treatment is most often used in cases of advanced cancer or those cases where tumour recurs following potentially curative surgical treatment.

🔑 KEY POINTS

- Although an elevated PSA and abnormal DRE may suggest prostate cancer, histological examination of a prostate biopsy is required for confirmation of the diagnosis and determination of important factors, which will affect prognosis and management decisions.
- Depending on the grade and stage of prostate cancer, management options range from active surveillance to surgery, radiotherapy and hormonal treatment.

CASE 51: A YOUNG MAN WITH A TESTICULAR LUMP

A 25-year-old man presents to the urology clinic with a nodule palpable in the left testis on self-examination. There is a history of groin injury during a game of rugby 3 weeks ago; however, the nodule is not painful.

Examination

A 1.5-cm, firm nodule is palpable at the lower pole of the left testis. There is no transillumi-nance, and the penis and scrotum are normal. There is no inguinal lymphadenopathy.

 INVESTIGATIONS

An ultrasound examination of the left testis demonstrates the lesion to be solid and with poorly defined margins. The right testis is normal, and there is no abdominal lymphadenopathy. Serum lactate dehydrogenase (LDH) is moderately elevated, while alpha-fetoprotein (AFP) and human chorionic gonadotropin (hCG) are normal.

? QUESTIONS

1. What is the differential diagnosis in this case?
2. What is the value of serum markers in the clinical management of this condition?
3. What pathological features are important in predicting the clinical outcome?

ANSWERS

A testicular nodule may represent any of the following lesions: a tumour, a cyst, a loculated hydrocele, or an inflammatory condition. A solid nodule with ill-defined borders on imaging is likely to be a malignant tumour, while that with a sharp circumscription is more likely to be benign; however, there are many exceptions to this rule. Cysts may also arise in the testis but more commonly in its vestigial remnants (appendix of testis and appendix of epididymis) and are benign, although they may enlarge and undergo torsion. Loculated hydrocele may develop secondary to trauma or inflammatory conditions. Fluid collections around the testis may be fluctuant and transilluminant on physical examination, and an ultrasound will confirm the fluid contents. Inflammatory conditions such as epididymo-orchitis (mumps, tuberculosis) are accompanied by systemic symptoms such as fever and a painful testicular mass. Syphilitic gumma may be painless, representing burnt-out disease (tertiary syphilis).

Serum tumour markers play an important role in the diagnosis, staging, risk stratification, and post-treatment monitoring of testicular cancer. On the other hand, serum markers are normal in testicular cysts and benign tumours such as Leydig cell adenoma.

Serum LDH is elevated in seminoma, but it is a relatively non-specific marker, as LDH is secreted by a number of other organs such as the liver. Serum AFP is elevated in yolk sac tumours, while hCG is produced in large quantities in a choriocarcinoma. Monitoring serum tumour marker levels after removal of the tumour is useful, as this would be accompanied by a steep decline in its serum levels, which may progressively rise again if there is tumour recurrence. Testicular tumours frequently occur in mixed forms so that one or more of these serum markers may be elevated.

Pathological examination of the testis following orchidectomy plays a key role in predicting clinical outcome. Malignant tumours (95%) are much more common than benign tumours. Broadly speaking, these are germ cell tumours and are subdivided into seminoma and non-seminomatous histological types. Seminoma is the most common subtype (80%), while embryonal carcinoma, yolk sac tumour, and choriocarcinoma are collectively referred to as non-seminomatous germ cell tumours (NSGCTs). Teratomas are another interesting subtype of testicular cancer characterised by the presence of somatic (epithelial and connective tissue) elements. NSGCTs may transform into the less aggressive teratoma following good response to chemotherapy.

Other adverse pathological features that influence clinical outcome include lymphovascular invasion, invasion of the rete testis, spermatic cord, peritoneal covering (tunica vaginalis), and scrotal skin. Ultrasound and CT scan are important in identifying metastases to lymph nodes and other organs such as lungs, liver, and bones.

Treatment of seminoma in the absence of these adverse features is orchidectomy and is curative in 80–85% cases. Adjuvant chemotherapy is required if adverse features are present or for NSGCT with markedly elevated serum tumour markers.

It is also important to remember that germ cell tumours may arise in an extratesticular location anywhere along the midline from the base of the skull to the sacrococcygeal tip.

🔑 **KEY POINTS**

- Testicular tumours are usually malignant, and the most common type is seminoma.
- Tumour markers and pathological features define the clinical outcome with a good chance of cure (80–85%) if these are favourable.
- Unfavourable histology and elevated tumour markers usually require adjuvant chemotherapy after orchidectomy.

CASE 52: HEAVY AND PAINFUL MENSTRUAL BLEEDING

A 40-year-old woman presents to her general practitioner complaining of increasingly heavy and painful menstrual bleeding. She denies any significant medical history and is taking no regular medication.

Examination

On examination the patient looks well, has a body mass index of 28, and no abnormality is found on abdominal examination.

 INVESTIGATIONS

Ultrasound pelvis: Several rounded, heterogeneous masses within the uterus, the largest of which measures 8 cm in diameter.

? QUESTIONS

1. What is the likely diagnosis?
2. The patient asks what the diagnosis means and what the treatment options are. How will you explain this to her?

ANSWERS

This patient has uterine fibroids, also known as leiomyomas. These are benign tumours of the muscle of the uterus (myometrium). Whereas fibroids are the most common benign tumours of the female genital tract (and of women in general), malignant tumours of the myometrium are rare and are called leiomyosarcomas. Fibroids typically present during the reproductive years, and most are asymptomatic. Others, depending on their size and location, may present with abdominal distension, abnormal menstrual bleeding (which in turn may lead to iron-deficiency anaemia), urinary frequency, pain during sexual intercourse or, rarely, infertility, which is associated more often with fibroids located immediately underneath the lining of the womb (endometrium). Malignant transformation is exceedingly rare, and most leiomyosar-comas are thought to arise de novo and not from leiomyomas.

Fibroids may be single or multiple and located anywhere within the uterus (subserosal, intra-mural, or submucosal), including the cervix, and can also be found in the uterine broad ligament. Although larger fibroids may be diagnosed by bimanual pelvic examination, the diagnosis is usually made through gynaecological ultrasound examination. Fibroids may also be diagnosed with magnetic resonance imaging (MRI), but neither imaging modality reliably distinguishes fibroids from their rare malignant counterpart. Larger fibroids may show changes such as infarction or haemorrhage, which makes this distinction more difficult.

Fibroids are monoclonal benign tumours, with nearly half of fibroids having a simple chromosomal abnormality. The aetiology is poorly understood, but factors that play a role in the development and growth of fibroids include a genetic predisposition, growth factors, and the effects and interplay of the hormones oestrogen and progesterone. Known risk factors include obesity, diabetes, hypertension, African descent and polycystic ovary syndrome.

Fibroids tend to shrink after menopause, when levels of oestrogen decrease. Therefore, it is typically only symptomatic fibroids in women in their reproductive years which require treatment. The treatment options may be medical (with drugs aimed at shrinking fibroids or controlling symptoms) or surgical (uterine artery embolisation, myomectomy or hysterectomy).

All fibroids need to be submitted for histological examination to exclude malignant change. Fibroids typically have a white or cream-coloured whorled cut surface and shell out with ease from the surrounding myometrium. Microscopically they consist of uniform smooth muscle cells arranged in bundles, with cigar-shaped nuclei and slender cytoplasmic processes. The presence of significant nuclear atypia, necrosis, and prominent mitotic activity will alert the pathologist that the fibroid may not be a leiomyoma, but its malignant counterpart, a leiomyosarcoma.

 KEY POINTS

- Fibroids (uterine leiomyomas) are the most common benign tumours of women and may present with vague abdominal symptoms, heavy menstrual bleeding, urinary symptoms or are commonly asymptomatic.
- Diagnosis is made by abdominal or bimanual pelvic examination or gynaecological ultrasonography.
- Management options depend on patient choice and size and location of fibroids, and may include medical, interventional radiological or surgical treatment.

CASE 53: ABNORMAL VAGINAL BLEEDING

A 35-year-old woman presents to her general practitioner complaining of post-coital vaginal bleeding and a vaginal discharge. She has no other medical history and has never had a cervical smear. She cohabits with a male partner and has no children.

Examination

General examination is within normal limits. The patient is referred for a cervical smear test, and on receipt of an abnormal result 10 days later, an urgent referral to the colposcopy service at her local hospital is made.

Colposcopic examination shows a firm mass distorting the cervix. Directed biopsies are obtained from the mass and submitted for pathological examination.

 INVESTIGATIONS

Cytological examination of the exfoliated superficial cervical epithelial cells sampled at the smear test shows severe squamous dyskaryosis and koilocytosis. The subsequent biopsy is reported as showing "invasive squamous cell carcinoma with associated CIN 3".

? QUESTIONS

1. What is the diagnosis?
2. What is the role of cervical screening?
3. How does this condition typically present?
4. What treatment options are available?

ANSWERS

The patient has cervical cancer. The most common type of cervical cancer is squamous cell carcinoma (approximately 85% of cervical cancers), with the rest being adenocarcinomas or adenosquamous carcinomas.

The vast majority of both squamous cell carcinomas and adenocarcinomas of the cervix are preceded by a precancerous lesion, known as cervical intraepithelial neoplasia (CIN) or cervical glandular intraepithelial neoplasia (CGIN), respectively. These precancerous lesions can be detected on smear tests of the cervix, commonly known as a Pap (Papanicolaou) smear, which is now being replaced by an improved method known as liquid-based cytology. As these precancerous lesions may exist in the non-invasive stage for many years, its timely diagnosis allows treatment to prevent progression to invasive carcinoma (although such progression is not invariably the case for all precancerous lesions).

Squamous cell carcinoma of the cervix may occur at any age from the late teens to old age but is most common in between the ages of 40 and 45 and approximately 10 years later than the peak incidence for high-grade intraepithelial neoplasia.

The National Health Service (NHS) cervical screening programme, which screens the highest-risk age group (25–49 years) every 3 years and those aged 50–64 every 5 years, has been highly successful, as evidenced by the marked decline in deaths from cervical cancer.

In almost all cases of cervical cancer, infection by human papillomavirus (HPV) is a necessary factor. This is a large group of viruses with several low-risk and high-risk types identified. Vaccines have been developed against two of the most important high-risk types (types 16 and 18), and HPV vaccination is currently being offered to certain groups of women and to girls aged 12–13 years. Smoking is a much less common risk factor for the development of cervical cancer, and the incidence of cervical cancer is higher in women with HIV disease.

The most common presenting symptoms of cervical cancer are abnormal vaginal bleeding or a vaginal discharge, but many cases are asymptomatic even at an advanced stage. Cervical precancers are most commonly asymptomatic, further demonstrating the importance of screening.

Treatment for precancerous lesions of the cervix, depending on the grade of abnormality, is typically local excision of the transformation zone of the cervix, known as an LLETZ, with more frequent follow-up by cervical smear following such treatment.

Treatment for invasive cervical carcinoma usually includes surgery (e.g., trachelectomy, in which the uterus and ovaries are not removed in order to preserve fertility, or hysterectomy) and in more advanced stages, radiotherapy and/or chemotherapy.

 KEY POINTS

- Cervical smear tests are an effective method of detecting the vast majority of cervical precancerous lesions so that preventative treatment can be offered.
- Cervical cancer is often asymptomatic, even in advanced stages, or may present with abnormal vaginal bleeding or a vaginal discharge.
- High-grade precancerous lesions and early stage invasive cancers are typically treated with surgical procedures in which fertility is retained.

CASE 54: A LUMP IN THE BREAST

A 33-year-old woman presents with a lump in her right breast that has been present for 2 weeks. It was detected on self-examination and has continued to enlarge. There is a history of ovarian cancer (mother), but not breast cancer, in her family.

Examination

A 2.5-cm-diameter lump is found in the upper outer quadrant of the right breast, which is hard and irregular but not fixed to the skin or to deeper tissue. There is also a palpable 1-cm lymph node in the right axilla. Examination of the contralateral breast and axilla is unremarkable.

 INVESTIGATIONS

- Ultrasound: Suspicious lump in right breast; axillary lymph node of normal echogenicity with a prominent vascular hilum.
- A core biopsy of the breast lump and fine needle aspiration (FNA) of the right axillary lymph node are performed.

? **QUESTIONS**

1. Is the history of ovarian cancer relevant in this patient?
2. Why are a core biopsy of the breast lump performed and FNA of the axillary lymph node?
3. What clinically useful information is provided by the tissue samples?

ANSWERS

The clinical and radiological features in this patient are suspicious of breast cancer. Breast cancer affects one in eight women (lifetime risk) in the UK. Screening for breast cancer by mammography or ultrasound begins at age 50 years in the UK, but 10 years earlier if there is a family history of breast or ovarian cancer. However, some patients may present with a tumour at an earlier age. Younger women tend to have ultrasound assessment, as they have more glandular tissue, whereas in older women, the breast undergoes fatty replacement, which makes them less dense and more amenable to mammographic assessment. Mammography will typically show a spiculated mass in breast cancer. However, it should be noted that mammography could miss palpable breast lumps and non-calcified lesions especially in the radio-dense breasts of premenopausal women. Between 10% and 40% of women who are found to have a mass by mammography will have breast cancer.

Core biopsy is the standard method of sampling a suspicious breast lump. This allows assessment of both invasive and in situ carcinoma; the latter is not reliably predicted by FNA and is important in clinical decision-making. However, FNA is preferred for targeting axillary nodes, as it is easier to direct a fine needle deep in the axilla under ultrasound guidance. It is less traumatic and poses a lower risk of accidentally puncturing deeper structures, including blood vessels and the pleura, compared to the larger core biopsy needle.

The core biopsy provides histological confirmation of whether the carcinoma invades the basement membrane and its subtype, such as ductal, lobular or mucinous carcinoma. Invasive ductal carcinoma is the most common subtype of breast cancer, accounting for around 75% of all breast cancer. It commonly metastasises to the axillary nodes and is associated with ductal carcinoma in situ (DCIS). Invasive lobular carcinoma shows a diffuse distribution in the breast, and hence is more likely to be multi-focal and bilateral.

Nuclear grading (1–3) of the tumour is also a prognostic marker, with higher grades of carcinoma being associated with a more aggressive clinical course. Tissue sampling also allows assessment of oestrogen and progesterone receptor expression by the tumour cells. Expression of these steroid receptors makes the tumour susceptible to hormone (anti-oestrogen) therapy and is associated with a better outcome compared to tumours that do not express these markers. Expression of c-erbB2 (Her2/neu) is also associated with better outcome and amenability to specific types of therapy in selected cases. The presence of lymphovascular invasion indicates the likelihood of spread of tumour cells beyond the breast, thereby conferring a poorer outlook. Without lymph node involvement, the 10-year disease-free survival is close to 70–80% but falls progressively with the number of involved nodes.

Clinical management of breast cancer includes using combinations of surgery, radiotherapy, hormonal therapy and systemic chemotherapy. In spite of good local control of disease, local and distant recurrences remain a problem in breast cancer, as tumour cells are believed to spread systemically early in the course of the disease.

🔑 **KEY POINTS**

- Breast carcinoma affects one in eight women, and a screening programme is available in the UK.
- Diagnosis relies on triple assessment by physical examination, radiology and biopsy.
- Despite advances in clinical management, local and distant recurrences remain a significant challenge.

CASE 55: LYMPH NODE ENLARGEMENT IN A YOUNG MAN

A 26-year-old Afro-Caribbean man is referred to the ear/nose/throat (ENT) clinic with progressively enlarging bilateral neck lumps. There is a history of mild, non-productive cough off and on but no fever or weight loss.

Examination

Examination of the neck reveals cervical lymphadenopathy with discrete, firm, non-tender nodes. There is no palpable lymphadenopathy in the axillae or groins. There is no clinical evidence of ENT infection.

INVESTIGATIONS

Fine needle aspiration (FNA) of the largest lymph node: groups of epithelioid cells in a reactive lymphoid background, with no evidence of necrosis or malignant cells.

QUESTIONS

1. What is the clinical differential diagnosis in this case?
2. What clinically useful information is available from the FNA?
3. What further investigations should be performed to confirm the diagnosis?

ANSWERS

The clinical differential diagnosis in this case includes tuberculosis (TB), sarcoidosis, and Hodgkin's lymphoma. Systemic symptoms such as fever and night sweats are seen in TB and lymphoma but are not reported by the patient. In TB, the lymph nodes are typically matted, while in Hodgkin's lymphoma these are rubbery and involve contiguous groups of nodes. Hence, the clinical history and investigation favours sarcoidosis by exclusion, but diagnosis requires histologic confirmation.

The FNA shows groups of epithelioid cells, which are modified macrophages with abundant cytoplasm and a footprint-shaped nucleus. Collections of epithelioid cells are called granulomata; hence the cytological diagnosis is granulomatous lymphadenitis. There is an accompanying mixed lymphoid population of mature and transformed lymphocytes. No necrosis is seen, which makes TB less likely, although this is not an essential feature. There is no evidence of Hodgkin's lymphoma in which Reed-Sternberg cells, mononuclear Hodgkin cells and eosinophils may be seen on FNA.

There are many possible causes for granulomatous inflammation. Infectious causes (besides *Mycobacteria*) include fungal infections such as *Histoplasma* and *Cryptococcus*. Non-infectious causes include inflammatory conditions such as Crohn's disease and sarcoidosis. Foreign bodies such as prosthetic implants and surgical suture material in tissues may also lead to formation of granulomata with giant cells.

Needle washings from the FNA should always be sent for detection of acid-fast bacilli (AFB) by direct demonstration on special stains such as Ziehl-Neelsen stain or auramine. Silver staining should be performed to look for fungal organisms. Microbiological culture should also be done, as AFB are not always detected on special stains.

In the given case, the FNA finding of non-necrotising granulomatous inflammation in a young man should prompt further investigations for sarcoidosis. If found to be elevated, the serum angiotensin-converting enzyme (ACE) level would suggest a diagnosis of sarcoidosis, since the enzyme is found in epithelioid cells forming granulomas. Serum calcium may also be elevated, since sarcoidal macrophages contain 1-α-hydroxylase, thereby leading to increased levels of 1,25-vitamin D, which is responsible for increasing calcium reabsorption from the gut as well as mobilisation from bone. Chest imaging (initially plain radiography and then CT) should be performed to look for pulmonary involvement, which is a common site of disease. Bilateral hilar lymphadenopathy is classically seen if the lungs are involved.

The aetiology of sarcoidosis is not well understood, but is believed to be due to dysregulation of the immune system after exposure to an as-yet-unidentified agent. The disease may affect any organ in the body, but often involves the lungs, producing a restrictive lung defect. Skin lesions may also be seen, with the combination of erythema nodosum, bilateral hilar lymphadenopathy, and arthralgia being called Löfgren's syndrome, a form of acute sarcoidosis. Systemic symptoms, such as fevers, night sweats, and weight loss, are also common.

Many patients with sarcoidosis do not require treatment, as the disease may remit spontaneously and often does so within 5 years. If patients are especially symptomatic, corticosteroids may be used. A small number of patients with pulmonary sarcoidosis may progress to progressive pulmonary fibrosis.

KEY POINTS

- Granulomata are collections of modified macrophages called epithelioid cells and are found as a specialised inflammatory response to certain agents, which may be infectious (e.g., *Mycobacteria*) or non-infectious (e.g., sarcoidosis)
- Sarcoidosis is a systemic illness, and investigations such as serum ACE levels, radiological investigations, and FNA are used in making the diagnosis.
- FNA is the first-line investigation for palpable lumps and can rapidly and accurately make a tissue diagnosis, avoiding the need for an excision biopsy.

CASE 56: AN ITCHY, BLEEDING MOLE ON THE BACK

A 64-year-old Caucasian male presents to his GP with darkening of a pre-existing mole on the back noticed by his wife whilst on holiday in the Bahamas. The patient complains that it is itchy and bleeds readily but attributes it to being out in the sun for long hours.

Examination

The mole measures 8 mm, having grown by 2 mm since it was last recorded by the GP a year ago. There is darkening of the lesion in the central part, and the edges appear irregular compared to the earlier examination. There is no palpable lymphadenopathy, and other moles on the body appear unchanged.

 INVESTIGATIONS

The GP refers the patient promptly to the dermatology clinic, where an excision biopsy of the lesion with a wide margin is performed.

? **QUESTIONS**

1. Why did the GP maintain a record of the patient's naevi?
2. What is the natural history of the progression of this lesion?
3. What are the clinical features that characterise this progression?

ANSWERS

Some kinds of pigmented lesions (dysplastic naevi) have a predisposition to malignant transformation, particularly if they are 5 mm or more in diameter in parts of the body not normally exposed to sunlight, if multiple lesions are present and if there is a family history of skin cancer. Regularly recording the appearances of a pigmented lesion and recognising the risk of development of melanoma in a dysplastic naevus indicates an alert GP.

Melanoma is a cancer of melanocytes, the pigmented cells in the skin, and is caused by injury to lightly pigmented skin by excessive exposure to ultraviolet (UV) radiation in sunlight. The change in colour of a pre-existing pigmented lesion with itching and bleeding and irregular margins on examination are indicators of transformation to melanoma.

Melanomas progress through a radial growth phase to a vertical growth phase. In the radial growth phase, the lesion expands horizontally within the epidermis and superficial dermis, often over a long period of time. Progression to the vertical phase is characterised by downward growth of the lesion into the deeper dermis and with absence of maturation of cells at the advancing front. During this phase, the lesion acquires the potential to metastasise through lymphovascular channels. The probability of this happening increases with increasing depth of invasion (Breslow thickness) by the melanoma cells. Mitotic activity indicates their aggressive potential. On the other hand, the presence of a lymphocytic reaction to the tumour is a favourable sign.

The ABCDE mnemonic aids in the diagnosis of melanoma:

- **A**symmetry—melanomas are likely to be irregular or asymmetrical
- **B**order—melanomas are more likely to have an irregular border with jagged edges
- **C**olour—melanomas tend to be variegated in colour and may have different shades, such as brown mixed with a black, red, pink, white or bluish tint
- **D**iameter—melanomas are usually more than 7 mm in diameter
- **E**volution—look for changes in the size, shape or colour of a mole

Most melanomas are less than 1 mm thick and are cured by complete excision, whilst thicker melanomas may spread to the regional lymph nodes. Fine needle aspiration (FNA) may confirm this spread, and surgical dissection of the lymph nodes may be necessary to clear the disease. Recurrences or spread of melanoma to other organs requires adjuvant treatment (BRAF-targeted chemotherapy, immunotherapy, and radiotherapy). Prevention is through protection from direct sunlight by use of appropriate clothing and the use of effective sunscreens.

 KEY POINTS

- Melanoma is a form of skin cancer, and UV radiation in sunlight (and sun beds) is the most important risk factor.
- Change in colour, irregularity of margins and itching are indicators of transformation to melanoma in a pre-existing naevus.
- The progression from radial to vertical growth phase marks the acquisition of metastatic potential of a melanoma.

CASE 57: BLOOD IN THE URINE OF AN ELDERLY MAN

A 68-year-old male presents to the urology outpatient clinic with a history of one episode of painless, frank haematuria a few days ago. He is a heavy smoker. On examination of the abdomen, he has ascites, which is confirmed on ultrasound.

? QUESTIONS

1. What is the most likely cause of the haematuria in this patient?
2. What investigations may be performed first based on the clinical data?
3. What is the definitive method of diagnosis of the suspected condition?

ANSWERS

Causes of haematuria include urinary tract calculi, infection, and malignancy (urothelial carcinoma). Given that the patient is a heavy smoker, a diagnosis of bladder cancer should be considered. Haematuria associated with calculi and infection may be accompanied by irritative symptoms and pain, while bladder cancer may be painless.

Urine cytology is an excellent test for detecting high-grade urothelial carcinoma. Twenty-five millilitres of voided urine is recommended, and a second morning voiding should be requested of the patient, as the first voiding of the day may show cellular degeneration in the bladder overnight. The sample is cytocentrifuged in the lab and a slide examined for malignant cells. If infection is suspected, an additional sample may also be sent to microbiology for culture and sensitivity.

In this patient, the ascitic fluid should also be examined for metastatic malignant cells from the bladder urothelial carcinoma. Fifty millilitres of serous fluid (ascitic, pleural, etc.) samples are recommended to improve the chances of picking up small numbers of malignant cells.

The definitive diagnosis of bladder cancer is made on cystoscopy and biopsy. Cystoscopy allows direct visualisation of the tumour, which may then be sampled for histological examination. Urothelial carcinoma may be papillary, flat (carcinoma in situ [CIS]), or invasive on histology. CIS and invasive carcinomas are high-grade, while the majority of papillary tumours tend to be low-grade, although a combination of low- and high-grade areas is common (tumour heterogeneity).

Histology also allows staging of urothelial carcinoma based on invasion into the lamina propria and muscularis propria (detrusor muscle). Non-invasive or those that only focally invade the lamina propria may be managed by transurethral resection and intravesical mitomycin or BCG (Bacillus Calmette-Guerin) instillation. Once the tumour invades the muscularis propria, radical treatment such as cystectomy or radiotherapy is necessary. More advanced cancers that have spread to lymph nodes or other sites may be considered for chemotherapy or immunotherapy.

 KEY POINTS

- Urine cytology is an excellent test for detecting high-grade urothelial carcinoma.
- The definitive diagnosis of bladder cancer is made on cystoscopy and biopsy.
- Histology also allows staging of urothelial carcinoma based on invasion into the lamina propria and muscularis propria (detrusor muscle).

CASE 58: THYROID DISEASE IN A YOUNG WOMAN

A 32-year-old woman presents with lethargy and mild weight gain. There are no abnormal clinical findings apart from a mildly enlarged thyroid gland. An ultrasound scan of the neck revealed a left-sided thyroid nodule on the background of diffuse vascularity. There was no cervical lymphadenopathy.

? QUESTIONS

1. What is the likely diagnosis based on the clinical data?
2. How is the diagnosis confirmed?
3. What are the complications of this condition?

ANSWERS

Autoimmune (Hashimoto's) thyroiditis is the most likely diagnosis and is the most common cause of hypothyroidism. Patients may present with cold intolerance, musculoskeletal pain, constipation, irregular menstrual periods, dry/thinning hair, depression, memory problems and a slowed heart rate. A history of thyroid disease in the family should be sought, as this is sometimes the case.

The diagnosis is confirmed by the detection of a high thyroid-stimulating hormone (TSH), low free T4 and presence of anti-thyroid antibodies, such as thyroid peroxidase antibodies (TPO) or thyroglobulin antibody. Ultrasound features include a diffusely hypoechoic thyroid gland, with increased vascularity on Doppler imaging.

Fine needle aspiration (FNA) of the thyroid nodule may reveal a lymphoplasmacytic infiltration with an excess of Hurthle (oncocytic) cells.

The treatment of Hashimoto's thyroiditis involves thyroid hormone replacement and management of the inflammatory process. Surgery may be indicated if the thyroid gland is enlarged and giving rise to obstructive symptoms such as shortness of breath, dysphagia or if the patient is unhappy with the cosmesis. These patients should be managed in a multidisciplinary setting that includes an endocrinologist and ear/nose/throat (ENT) surgeon.

Long-term complications of hypothyroidism include high cholesterol, myxoedema, heart disease, complications during pregnancy and development of thyroid lymphoma. This tends to be a B-cell lymphoma that presents in a female, elderly patient, with a rapidly enlarging thyroid mass.

KEY POINTS

- Autoimmune (Hashimoto's) thyroiditis is the most common cause of hypothyroidism.
- The diagnosis is confirmed by the detection of a high TSH, low free T4, and presence of anti-thyroid antibodies.
- FNA of the thyroid nodule may reveal a lymphoplasmacytic infiltration with an excess of Hurthle (oncocytic) cells.

Section 3
HAEMATOLOGY

CASE 59: SHORTNESS OF BREATH AND HEARTBURN

A 52-year-old gentleman presents to his GP complaining of shortness of breath on exertion and fatigue, which has been worsening for the past 3 months. During a systemic enquiry, the patient reveals that his previously uninvestigated heartburn and indigestion have recently become increasingly bothersome, especially at night. This is unabated by over-the-counter antacids. The patient also admits to using regular ibuprofen for long-term knee pain. He denies any change in weight, bowel habit or appetite. He has drunk 30 units of alcohol per week for the past 20 years, but does not smoke. He attributes his symptoms to the stress caused by looking after his disabled son.

Examination

The patient is apyrexial but looks pale. His heart rate is 90, regular rhythm. The GP also notes angular stomatitis. Examinations of his cardiorespiratory and abdominal systems are unremarkable.

INVESTIGATIONS

	Haemoglobin	101
	White cell count	7.1
	Red cell count	6.0
	Platelets	500
	Mean corpuscular volume	75
	Mean cell haemoglobin	20
	Thyroid-stimulating hormone	2
Iron profile		
	Serum iron	9
	Serum ferritin	10
	Total iron binding capacity	77
	Transferrin saturation	10%

B_{12} and folate levels both were normal.

Urinalysis: Negative for blood, protein, and glucose.

Peripheral blood film shows hypochromic microcytic cells and pencil-shaped poikilocytes.

QUESTIONS

1. What is the most likely diagnosis?
2. What further investigations would you arrange?
3. Would you arrange a blood transfusion for this patient?

ANSWERS

This patient's haematological indices suggest anaemia (low haemoglobin level), with microcytic red cells demonstrating low MCV (reflecting reduced average red cell size) and MCH (reduced number of haemoglobin molecules per red cell).

The iron profile suggests a deficiency of serum iron, associated with a reduction in the amount of iron storage (ferritin) and an increase in the body's attempts to bind to serum iron (TIBC). Both serum iron and ferritin levels are affected by other conditions—for example, ferritin increases with liver disease and infection. Hence, unless the patient does not have any other pathology, their levels may not give an accurate assessment of the iron status in the body. Haematologists tend to rely more on transferrin saturation for giving an accurate assessment.

Usually the body absorbs less than 10% of dietary iron via the duodenum. Absorption is impaired by tea and alkaline foods such as vegetables. During deficiency, an increase in iron absorption is concomitant with a rise in transferrin, which acts to carry iron to developing red cells in the bone marrow. A high level of transferrin distinguishes iron deficiency from other causes of anaemia.

The peripheral blood smear shows hypochromic (pale) red blood cells. There are also long, pencil-shaped red cells, typically seen in iron deficiency. All of these features point towards iron deficiency as a cause of this man's anaemia. The raised platelet count is also a recognised feature of iron-deficiency anaemia.

A differential diagnosis would include beta thalassaemia trait because this also produces anaemia with low MCV. Usually beta thalassaemia trait would demonstrate raised haemoglobin A2 (HbA2). Sideroblastic anaemia can present with microcytic, normocytic, or macrocytic anaemia. However, the levels of iron and ferritin may be raised, with a normal TIBC. Bone marrow biopsy would demonstrate ring sideroblasts, which are erythroblasts in which the nucleus is encircled by rings of mitochondria containing iron deposits.

Iron deficiency is the most common cause of anaemia worldwide. It takes several years for dietary deficiency of iron to manifest. The more common causes are chronic blood loss from the heavy menstrual bleeding in women and bleeding from the gastrointestinal system in men and women. Iron can also be lost through the skin, as seen in exfoliative dermatitis. Other causes include increased demand for iron as seen in newborns, adolescents and pregnant and lactating women. Gluten enteropathy and a gastrectomy can also predispose to iron deficiency.

Occasionally patients (usually children) with iron deficiency will exhibit pica, which is an appetite for non-nutritive substances like crushed ice, paper or chalk. This disappears upon correction of iron levels.

Acute blood loss presents with a normochromic normocytic (as opposed to hypochromic microcytic) anaemia and reticulocytosis because plasma volume is able to re-expand over the course of 3–7 days. However there are several clinical indicators of chronic blood loss in this patient's history. These include worsening heartburn and indigestion, a long-term history of non-steroid anti-inflammatory drug (ibuprofen) use and high alcohol intake. Gastrointestinal (GI) lesions are commonly associated with bleeding and iron deficiency. Further investigations in this patient included both upper GI tract endoscopy and a colonoscopy. This revealed gastritis and a duodenal ulcer. Biopsies showed positivity for *Helicobacter pylori* infection.

Blood transfusion is not indicated for this patient. Unfortunately, many clinicians tend to rush and give a blood transfusion when it is not indicated. A low haemoglobin level is not on its own an indication for blood transfusion. A healthy patient with iron deficiency should be expected to recover his normal haemoglobin levels with adequate iron supplements. Oral ferrous sulphate is available, and if not tolerated, other products such as ferrous fumarate can be an alternative. If oral iron is not effective, intravenous iron can be given and is usually very effective in treating iron deficiency.

A common threshold for transfusion is a haemoglobin level of 80 g/L or less, but this in itself is not an absolute indication. Young patients with iron deficiency and a haemoglobin level of less than 80 g/L who are not symptomatic are expected to recover well with iron supplements. The patient's symptoms—chest pain or dizziness—and clinical signs—low BP and tachycardia—should be taken into consideration when deciding on whether to give a blood transfusion. (Note: Patients with a history of ischaemic heart disease usually need a higher level of haemoglobin. Therefore, the haemoglobin level may need to be maintained at 100 g/L or higher.)

 KEY POINTS

- Iron-deficiency anaemia is commonly caused by dietary deficiencies, but all patients need to be assessed for possible blood loss because of a GI lesion, and if indicated, appropriate investigations should be arranged.
- In practice a low transferrin saturation is a good indicator of iron deficiency in the body.
- Blood transfusion should not be given based on low haemoglobin levels alone: the patient's symptoms and signs need to be taken into consideration.

CASE 60: RAISED WHITE CELL COUNT IN AN ASYMPTOMATIC INDIVIDUAL

A healthy 65-year-old man undergoes routine blood tests as part of a 'well-man screen' by his GP. His past medical history includes appendicectomy and inguinal hernia repair. He does not take any regular medications.

Examination

Cardiovascular and respiratory examinations are normal. He has no organomegaly or lymphadenopathy.

🔍 INVESTIGATIONS

Haemoglobin	142
White cell count	20.1
Neutrophils	5
Lymphocytes	14
Platelets	350
Mean cell volume	86

The remainder of his blood tests were unremarkable, including urea and electrolytes, liver function, thyroid function and prostate specific antigen (PSA).

The patient is referred to the haematology clinic, where further investigations are performed, including a blood film (Figure 60.1) and immunophenotyping.

Immunophenotype of lymphocytes: CD5/19/20/23+ve and CD79b negative.

The haematologist elects to adopt a 'watch-and-wait' treatment strategy and discharges the man to receive follow-up blood tests with his GP. The blood tests do not show significant changes over time.

Three years later, the patient develops increasing fatigue. On examination, there is conjunctival pallor and mild scleral icterus but no lymphadenopathy or organomegaly. Direct antiglobulin test is positive. A repeat blood test is arranged, which shows:

Haemoglobin	98
White cell count	30.1
Neutrophils	5
Lymphocytes	24
Platelets	250
Mean cell volume	86

❓ QUESTIONS

1. What are the common causes of lymphocytosis?
2. Based on the initial blood results and the blood film, what is the likely diagnosis?
3. Explain how the results from the latest blood tests (at 3 years) relate to the patient's underlying diagnosis.
4. What are the indications of treatment for this condition?

DOI: 10.1201/9781003242697-63

ANSWERS

The initial full blood count shows a lymphocytic leucocytosis. Causes of lymphocytosis include:

- Infection, both acute (e.g., infectious mononucleosis, mumps, herpes simplex/zoster, and HIV) and chronic (tuberculosis and syphilis)
- Inflammation
- Chronic lymphoid leukaemias, most commonly chronic lymphocytic leukaemia (CLL)
- Acute lymphoblastic leukaemia (ALL)
- Non-Hodgkin's lymphoma

In the absence of symptoms (such as features of infection) and signs (such as lymphadenopathy and organomegaly), and with normal thyroid function, the most likely diagnosis in this case is CLL. This is corroborated by the blood film shown in Figure 60.1, which shows increased numbers of small, mature lymphocytes with scant cytoplasm. As these cells are fragile, they may be disrupted in the process of making smears, giving rise to 'smudge cells' that are seen in film. Immunophenotyping is required to confirm the diagnosis of CLL, and the phenotype of CD5, CD20 and CD23 positivity is characteristic of CLL.

CLL is the most common leukaemia in the Western world. Typically, it is picked up via an incidental lymphocytosis in an asymptomatic individual. Diagnosis requires an absolute lymphocytosis of at least 5×10^9/L and an appropriate lymphocyte immunophenotype. Common cytogenetic abnormalities in CLL include deletions of chromosomes 11, 13 and 17 (del 11q, del 13q, del 17p), as well as trisomy 12. About 50% of cases also show evidence of somatic hypermutation of the immunoglobulin heavy-chain gene (IGVH).

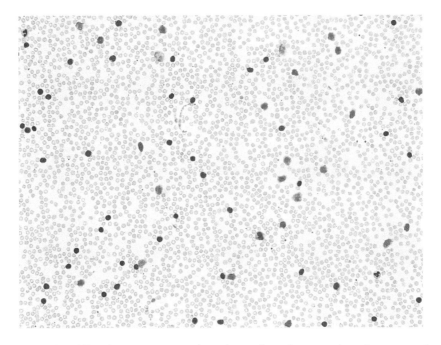

Figure 60.1 Blood film showing increased numbers of small, mature lymphocytes with scant cytoplasm. Being fragile, they have been disrupted in the process of making smears, giving rise to 'smudge cells'.

The disease is staged according to the Binet classification. Typically, patients with Binet stage A disease require no immediate treatment. Symptomatic stage B and all stage C patients receive chemotherapy. Options for treatment include conventional chemotherapy combined with immunotherapy, e.g., fludarabine, cyclophosphamide and rituximab (FCR) or more targeted treatments, e.g., ibrutinib (inhibitor of BTK enzyme) or venetoclax (inhibitor of BCL2). The aim of the treatment is generally disease control rather than cure. Younger patients with refractory disease may be considered for allogeneic stem cell transplantation, which is potentially curative but has a significant morbidity and mortality rate.

The patient's blood results at 3 years highlight an important complication of CLL. They show a normocytic anaemia (as well as a marked lymphocytosis). The latter represents progression of CLL, but the absence of neutropenia and thrombocytopenia suggests that marrow infiltration is not severe. However, taken together with the positive direct antiglobulin test (DAT), the most likely explanation for the anaemia is haemolytic (immune mediated). Autoimmune haemolytic anaemia is sometimes seen in CLL as a result of autoantibody generation by lymphocytes against red blood cells. This produces pallor (due to anaemia) and icterus (as a result of increased destruction of red cells, leading to an unconjugated hyperbilirubinaemia).

Not all patients require treatment. Adverse prognostic features include stage B or C disease at diagnosis, male gender, rapid lymphocyte doubling time (<1 year), presence of del 11q and del 17p, TP53 mutation, trisomy 12, positivity for CD38 expression and high ZAP-70 expression. There is also a possibility that CLL may transform into a high-grade lymphoma, diffuse large B-cell lymphoma or Hodgkin's lymphoma (a so-called Richter transformation).

 KEY POINTS

- CLL is the most common form of leukaemia in the Western world.
- CLL is a lymphoproliferative disorder of mature lymphocytes and typically presents as an incidental finding in asymptomatic patients.
- Treatment is not always indicated, but careful monitoring is required.
- Autoimmune haemolytic anaemia is a known complication of CLL, caused by auto-antibody production by diseased lymphocytes against red blood cells.

CASE 61: WORSENING FATIGUE AND BLEEDING GUMS

A 35-year-old woman presents to her GP with fatigue. She visited the GP surgery 4 weeks ago with the same problem. At that time all of her routine blood tests (including thyroid function tests) were reported as normal. Today she has noticed some gum bleeding while brushing her teeth. She does not have a cough, urinary symptoms, weight loss or fevers. She has no significant past medical history.

Examination

Her observations are normal. She appears pale. Examinations of her cardiovascular, respiratory and abdominal systems are normal.

INVESTIGATIONS

Haemoglobin	89
White cell count	1.9
Neutrophils	0.9
Lymphocytes	0.8
Platelets	13
Mean corpuscular volume	106
Sodium	141
Potassium	5.0
Urea	5.0
Creatinine	70
Bilirubin	20
Aspartate aminotransferase	70
Alkaline phosphatase	160
C-reactive protein	13

Her blood film is shown in Figure 61.1.

QUESTIONS

1. What is the diagnosis?
2. What other tests do you need to arrange?
3. What is your management plan for this patient?

ANSWERS

The patient has pancytopenia with blast cells in the circulation consistent with a diagnosis of acute leukaemia. The patient is lethargic due to the anaemia. She is also bleeding because of low platelets. She is at increased risk of infections due to neutropenia. Blast cells are immature cells that turn into mature blood cells in the bone marrow. In acute leukaemia, an arrest in the maturation process keeps these cells at their early non-functioning stage, and they begin to divide rapidly; the increased proliferation occupies space in the bone marrow, thereby disturbing the normal haemopoiesis and eventually leading to pancytopenia.

The blast cells eventually leak out into the circulation, and they can be seen on a peripheral blood film. They are usually large in size (causing a higher MCV reading in the full blood count) with an open chromatin appearance. They are also light in colour compared to the nuclei of mature cells, which are smaller and darker. Blast cells have a high nucleus-to-cytoplasmic ratio (a large nucleus in scanty cytoplasm).

Distinguishing between acute myeloid leukaemia (AML) and acute lymphoid leukaemia (ALL) using morphological features alone is possible; however, this is not always easy. More detailed analysis of the cells is usually carried out to determine the exact diagnosis

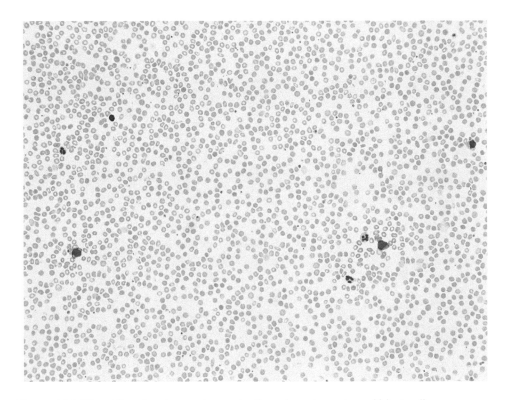

Figure 61.1 Blood film showing neutropenia, thrombocytopenia and blast cells.

Other investigations will include a bone marrow biopsy. The biopsy provides tissue that can be examined for:

- Further morphological assessment, as the percentage of blast cells would be much higher in the bone marrow. The general haemopoietic status of the bone marrow can also be assessed.
- Immunophenotyping studies to test the CD markers on the blast cells, which should provide a more accurate assessment of their nature.
- Cytogenetic studies, as certain chromosomal abnormalities are associated with adverse prognosis, which will influence treatment options (e.g., whether to offer the patient stem cell transplant or not).
- Molecular studies, e.g., FLT3 mutation in AML or BCR-ABL fusion in ALL.

Clotting studies are important. Variants such as acute promyelocytic leukaemia (APML) are associated with disseminated intravascular coagulation (DIC), which can be life threatening, especially with a very low platelet count.

The patient is neutropenic, so she needs close observation. Fever should initiate septic screening and administration of intravenous antibiotics as a matter of urgency (according to local neutropenic sepsis guidelines).

This patient would also benefit from a platelet transfusion. Haematologists usually aim for a level of greater than $20 \times 10^9/L$, especially if the patient is septic. This patient's deranged liver function tests may represent leukaemic infiltration or another pathology of the liver. Blood tests for a liver screen and an abdominal ultrasound scan should be arranged.

Acute leukaemia can infiltrate other organs, especially the central nervous system (CNS) in ALL. A careful screening of the patient's symptoms, asking her about headaches and clinical examination to exclude neurological signs, is essential. If there is any suspicion of CNS involvement, a CT scan of the brain is needed, and a lumbar puncture should be performed to evaluate the cerebrospinal fluid (CSF) for the presence of leukaemic cells.

The initial treatment will be chemotherapy, but an allogenic stem cell transplant may be required. Therefore, it would be useful to know whether she has siblings who can be tested as potential future donors of stem cells. Otherwise, a search for a matched unrelated donor will be required to find suitable human leukocyte antigen (HLA)–matched stem cells.

 KEY POINTS

- Acute leukaemia is a medical emergency that needs to be excluded in any patient with an isolated cytopenia or pancytopenia.
- Neutropenic sepsis is a serious complication of acute leukaemia. It can occur at presentation or during treatment and needs to be treated urgently with intravenous antibiotics without any delay.
- The exact treatment of acute leukaemia will depend on the type of leukaemia, which can be determined through immunophenotyping, cytogenetics and molecular studies.

CASE 62: BURNING URINE AND AN ABNORMAL CLOTTING SCREEN

A 45-year-old woman presents to the emergency department with pain in her left loin and painful micturition. Her symptoms started 2 days ago with increased frequency of passing urine, and now she has developed a burning sensation. She has no past medical history, and she is not allergic to any medications.

Examination

She has fever of 38.3°C, pulse 120, BP 90/60, peripheral oxygen saturations 96% on room air. Cardiovascular and respiratory examinations are normal. Abdominal examination shows tenderness worse over the left kidney. Urine dipstick is positive for blood, leukocytes and nitrites.

INVESTIGATIONS

Haemoglobin	115
White cell count	33.0
Neutrophils	28.0
Lymphocytes	5.0
Platelets	35
Mean corpuscular volume	80
Sodium	148
Potassium	5.9
Urea	20.0
Creatinine	300
Bilirubin	20
Aspartate aminotransferase	70
Alkaline phosphatase	160
C-reactive protein	200
Prothrombin time	30
Activated partial thromboplastin time	50
Fibrinogen	0.5
D-dimer	600

? QUESTIONS

1. Based on the history and blood results, what is the most likely diagnosis?
2. What is your management plan for this patient?
3. What are the possible complications of this syndrome?

ANSWERS

The patient has urinary symptoms, positive urine dipstick, signs of sepsis (fever, tachycardia and hypotension) and raised serum inflammatory markers. These are all suggestive of urinary sepsis.

She also has acute renal failure (assuming she had a normal baseline) and deranged clotting. She has prolonged clotting times (PT and APTT) and low fibrinogen. She also has elevated D-dimers, which are products of fibrin degradation (giving an indication of fibrin formation). These clotting abnormalities are features of disseminated intravascular coagulation (DIC).

DIC is a syndrome that is characterised by loss of control of intravascular activation of coagulation. The hallmark of DIC is the widespread activation of thrombin, and hence thrombosis, that leads to excessive consumption of coagulation factors and platelets, and as a consequence leads to excessive bleeding. The simultaneous thrombosis and bleeding, in association with the activation of the inflammatory cascade, causes widespread organ damage and high mortality.

Associated organ damage can precipitate the abnormalities in DIC: renal failure could impair platelet function, liver failure decreases synthesis of clotting factors and endothelial dysfunction depletes nitric oxide from the circulation, which leads to constant platelet activation.

Several conditions are associated with DIC:

- Sepsis
- Trauma (head injury, burns, fat embolism)
- Malignancy
- Obstetric complications (placental abruption, pre-eclampsia)
- Pancreatitis

The best treatment in DIC is to treat the cause. In the case of this patient, the urinary sepsis was treated with intravenous antibiotics and fluids. Supportive therapy with blood products is also needed:

- Platelet transfusion to keep the platelet count greater than $50 \times 10^9/L$ if there is a high risk of bleeding.
- Fresh frozen plasma (FFP) is a source of clotting factors, except fibrinogen. The adult dose is 15 mL/kg, which is approximately equivalent to four units of FFP.
- Cryoprecipitate or fibrinogen concentrate should be given to keep the fibrinogen level greater than 1.5.
- Prothrombin complex concentrate (PCC) could be considered, and in severe bleeding recombinant (r) factor VIIa may be advised. However, these special products need to be discussed with the haematology team prior to their use.

Widespread thrombosis in the microcirculation of organs leads to ischaemia and possible permanent damage in the kidneys, liver, spleen, lungs and brain.

 KEY POINTS

- DIC is a syndrome that can be triggered by several conditions, including renal and liver failure.
- It is characterised by simultaneous thrombosis and bleeding as a result of consumption of clotting factors.
- The best treatment is to treat the cause and use supportive blood products.

CASE 63: HEADACHES, BLURRED VISION AND ITCHING

A 64-year-old man presents to his GP with headaches and blurred vision. He has been complaining of these symptoms for a few weeks. He has no neck stiffness and no vomiting, and the headaches are not worse on straining. The only other thing he has noticed recently is severe itching all over his skin, especially after taking a bath. He is not a smoker, he drinks occasionally and the only medication he takes is simvastatin.

Examination

The patient has normal observations and oxygen saturation of 99% on room air. The GP noticed a general plethora and dilated vessels in both conjunctiva. Cardiovascular and respiratory examinations were normal. He had a palpable spleen approximately 5 cm below the costal margins. Neurological examination is normal.

INVESTIGATIONS

Haemoglobin	180
Packed cell volume	0.62
White cell count	7.0
Neutrophils	5.0
Lymphocytes	1.0
Platelets	700
Mean corpuscular volume	80
Sodium	142
Potassium	5.0
Urea	4.0
Creatinine	99
Bilirubin	10
Aspartate aminotransferase	50
Alkaline phosphatase	110
C-reactive protein	6

QUESTIONS

1. What is the most likely diagnosis?
2. What other tests would you arrange to confirm the diagnosis?
3. What is your management plan?

ANSWERS

The patient has erythrocytosis (a high haemoglobin level), thrombocytosis (a high platelet level) and polycythaemia (a high haematocrit and packed cell volume [PCV]). Given his presentation and his splenomegaly, this is most likely polycythaemia vera (PV).

PV is a haematological disorder with expansion of all three major myeloid cell lineages: red blood cells, neutrophils, and platelets. The majority of patients have a mutation in the tyrosine kinase JAK2, the main function of which is to stimulate erythropoiesis. The most common mutation is V167F, followed by mutation in exon 12.

In PV, erythropoiesis is autonomous as a consequence of these mutations and does not depend on the erythropoietin (EPO) hormone. In fact, EPO levels are reduced in PV.

True polycythaemia needs to be distinguished from apparent polycythaemia. The former is a true increase in total red cell mass, while the latter is caused by a reduction in plasma volume. True polycythaemia may be primary (either a clonal disorder such as PV or the result of an inherited defect either in EPO receptors or the red cell precursors) or secondary. Secondary polycythaemia is best divided according to whether it is associated with hypoxia or not. Conditions with systemic hypoxia, such as lung disease, heavy smoking and congenital cyanotic heart disease, may all cause secondary polycythaemia. Other conditions, without hypoxia, may also cause polycythaemia:

- Elevated levels of EPO due to either inherited conditions or to renal or liver disease
- Endocrine conditions such as Cushing's disease and Conn's syndrome

PV usually presents with neurological symptoms, similar to the patient in this case. Such symptoms are due to increased viscosity of the blood and the sluggish cerebral circulation. Pruritus occurs in almost 25% of patients. Thrombotic events, either arterial or venous, especially in splenic vessels, are serious complications of PV and can be the presenting feature in previously undiagnosed patients. Many patients also are diagnosed incidentally on a routine blood test.

To confirm the diagnosis, the following are required:

- JAK2 mutation screen (for V617F and exon 12 mutations).
- EPO levels to exclude secondary polycythaemia.
- Abdominal ultrasound scan to measure the spleen and to search for an abdominal lesion that may be responsible for high EPO levels.
- If there is a possibility of hypoxia or lung disease, then arterial blood gas measurement to measure oxygenation levels. Carboxyhaemoglobin can be tested in heavy smoking as well.
- If these tests do not confirm the diagnosis, then other tests can be arranged, e.g., red cell mass studies and high-affinity haemoglobins.

Venesection to reduce the PCV to less than 0.45 is an effective way to improve a patient's symptoms and reduce the risk of thrombosis. Patients initially undergo weekly venesection until their PCV is below 0.45, after which at 4- to 6-week and then 2- to 3-month intervals.

If venesection is not effective or not tolerated by the patient (dizziness is a common side effect), cytoreductive therapy can be considered. Hydroxycarbamide is a common option. Patients with significant thrombocytosis may benefit from aspirin.

KEY POINTS

- PV is a clonal disorder affecting all three myeloid lineages (haemoglobin, neutrophils and platelets).
- JAK2 mutation is detected in the majority of cases and needs to be tested in any patient with unusual thrombosis, e.g., splenic vein thrombosis.
- Venesection is an effective treatment for PV.

CASE 64: A PAINFUL ARM AND A LARGE SPLEEN

A 5-year-old boy is brought to the emergency department by his mother. They are originally from Nigeria and have recently arrived in the country. The boy is complaining of pain in his right forearm. He has no diarrhoea or vomiting. He has no history of injury or falls. His mother reports that he has never seen a doctor before and he is the only child in the family. She recalls that the only other symptom he had was a runny nose a few days ago.

Examination

His right forearm is tender, but not hot or swollen. The tip of the spleen is palpable. His cardiorespiratory examination is normal. He is also noted to be limping. He is not complaining of any pain in his feet, but neurological assessment of his legs showed mild weakness in his left leg and increased reflexes.

INVESTIGATIONS

Haemoglobin	60
White cell count	20.0
Platelets	600
Mean corpuscular volume	80
Bilirubin	40
Aspartate aminotransferase	100
Alkaline phosphatase	300
C-reactive protein	100

Urea and electrolytes unremarkable.

His blood film is shown in Figure 64.1.

QUESTIONS

1. What does the blood film show?
2. Why does the child have pain in his right forearm?
3. What other tests would you arrange?
4. What is your management plan?
5. What is the explanation of his limping?

ANSWERS

The blood film shows numerous sickle cells, which is likely to represent homozygous inheritance of sickle haemoglobin (Hb-S). This child has sickle cell disease, which is a type of inherited chronic haemolytic anaemia.

His blood tests confirm anaemia and show an inflammatory response: elevated white cell count, platelets, and C-reactive protein. Given that he is presenting with coryzal symptoms, it is likely that he has an infection. His deranged liver function tests could reflect the underlying infection, but it is more likely that haemolysis has caused his elevated bilirubin and low haemoglobin level.

Haemolysis is a chronic process in sickle cell disease, but during an infection, acute-on-chronic haemolysis takes place. It is vital that for such patients the baseline haemoglobin is known. In the case of this child who arrived recently from Nigeria, where sickle cell is commonly inherited, it seems that his mother is not aware of his diagnosis. He is likely to have been missed on screening when he was born.

Hb-S is caused by a single nucleotide change in the beta-globin chain that results in the substitution of valine for glutamic acid. This increases the tendency for Hb-S to polymerise in de-oxygenated conditions. This intracellular polymerisation gives the red blood cells the elongated sickle shape (Figure 64.1). These cells have reduced deformability, and their flow through small capillaries increases blood viscosity, causing vaso-occlusion, hypoxia and bone infarction. Bone pain is the most common symptom of a vaso-occlusive crisis and can be very severe.

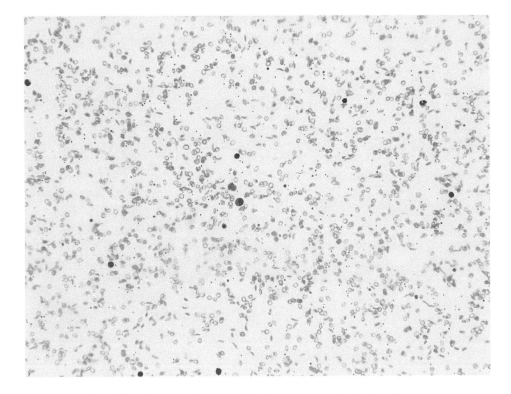

Figure 64.1 Blood film showing elongated, sickle-shaped red blood cells.

A septic screen should be performed that includes a blood culture, urine microscopy, culture and sensitivity, chest radiograph and a viral swab from his nasal discharge. A plain radiograph of his right forearm will help exclude bone injury and osteomyelitis. The patient also needs to have a group-and-save sample, with extended phenotype matching to be performed by the blood transfusion lab. An ultrasound scan of the abdomen to measure the size of the spleen and exclude any other liver pathology is necessary. Most sickle cell disease patients have atrophic spleens because of recurrent vaso-occlusion and infarction, which leaves them with non-functioning spleens. They need vaccination against encapsulated bacteria, so a vaccination every 5 years against pneumococcal bacteria is required, as well as annual influenza vaccination. Also, they have chronic haemolytic anaemia, so they need regular folic acid to maintain a supply to the newly formed red blood cells.

This patient is likely suffering from a painful (vaso-occlusive) sickle cell crisis precipitated by a viral infection. Pain needs to be controlled. The first line is regular paracetamol and non-steroidal anti-inflammatory drugs (NSAIDs). If the mother already tried them, then codeine phosphate could be given. Some patients with sickle cell disease have severe painful episodes, which can be quite frequent and require hospital admission. Morphine should be used promptly for such patients.

In addition to analgesia, patients must have adequate hydration and oxygenation because the polymerisation of Hb-S is influenced by the oxygenation status and dehydration. Start intravenous fluids if oral hydration is not adequate.

If there is any suspicion of bacterial infection, antibiotics must be started. Haemoglobin baseline level varies between patients with sickle cell disease, but they tend to have lower levels than the rest of the population. This patient's haemoglobin level is borderline low, and it needs to be monitored closely. Most physicians would transfuse if it drops below 60 g/L in sickle cell disease. This needs to be anticipated, and thus a sample is usually sent to the blood transfusion lab on admission. Importantly, since some of these patients need recurrent blood transfusions over their lifetime, the laboratory would usually give extended phenotype matching blood units. This means they are matched not only for the ABO and RhD blood groups but for other blood groups as well. This is to reduce the risk of developing antibodies against these other blood groups, which would lead to difficulty in finding suitable units of blood to transfuse the patient in the future.

One of the severe complications of sickle cell disease is stroke, which can be silent in children. This patient needs an MRI of the brain to exclude this and a referral to a paediatric haematologist for long-term follow-up and a secondary prevention programme to protect against further brain damage.

 KEY POINTS

- Sickle cell disease is an inherited chronic haemolytic anaemia.
- Infections can precipitate painful episodes from vaso-occlusion, and they need prompt treatment.
- Other long-term complications of the disease need to be addressed: chronic haemolytic state, vaccination and reducing the risk of cerebrovascular disease.
- Psychological support and family education are vital in such chronic conditions.

CASE 65: A RASH ON THE THIGHS

A 34-year-old woman presents to her GP with a rash on her thighs, which appeared this morning. She started noticing it following 2 days of coryzal symptoms.

Following a quick assessment, the GP suspects meningitis and administers intramuscular benzylpenicillin and refers the patient to the local emergency department. Upon arrival, the doctors take a more detailed history. She has no photophobia or neck stiffness, and apart from being worried about the rash, she is otherwise well. She also remembers some gum bleeding from the night before while she was brushing her teeth. Her family history reveals several relatives with autoimmune disease.

Examination

She is not febrile, and cardiovascular and respiratory examinations are normal. She has no palpable spleen, liver, or lymph nodes. The rash is purpuric and does not blanch on stretching the skin. Joint examination is unremarkable.

🔍 INVESTIGATIONS

Haemoglobin	125
White cell count	12.0
Neutrophils	1.0
Lymphocytes	7.0
Platelets	8
Mean corpuscular volume	80
C-reactive protein	23

Blood film is shown in Figure 65.1.

❓ QUESTIONS

1. What are the two most likely differential diagnoses?
2. How would you describe the findings in her blood film? What abnormal cells are you looking for?
3. Does this patient need platelet transfusion?
4. What is your management plan?

ANSWERS

Blood results show thrombocytopenia and mild neutropenia with lymphocytosis. The top two differential diagnoses are leukaemia, which affects normal haemopoiesis and causes cytopenia by the rapid division of abnormal leukaemia cells in the bone marrow. The other main differential diagnosis is primary immune thrombocytopenia (ITP), previously known as idiopathic thrombocytopenic purpura, which typically causes low platelets and sometimes neutropenia if there is a concurrent viral illness or autoimmune disease.

To exclude leukaemia, a blood film is usually examined for blast cells, which are cells with abnormal maturation. This blood film (Figure 65.1) does not show blast cells. Instead it confirms thrombocytopenia, neutropenia, and giant platelets at the centre of the film.

This patient has ITP, which is an autoimmune condition characterised by low platelets and tendency to bleed. It was initially thought to be a condition caused purely by autoantibodies against platelets leading to opsonisation and premature destruction in the reticuloendothelial system. However, recently a deeper understanding of the pathophysiology has shown that in fact other mechanisms are involved.

Autoantibodies opsonise megakaryocytes, which are the cells of the bone marrow that synthesise platelets. This has an inhibitory effect of their growth and platelet release and induces apoptosis. Relatively low levels of free thrombopoietin (TPO), the hormone that drives platelet production, might also be contributing to low levels of platelets, as may T-cell–directed lysis of platelets.

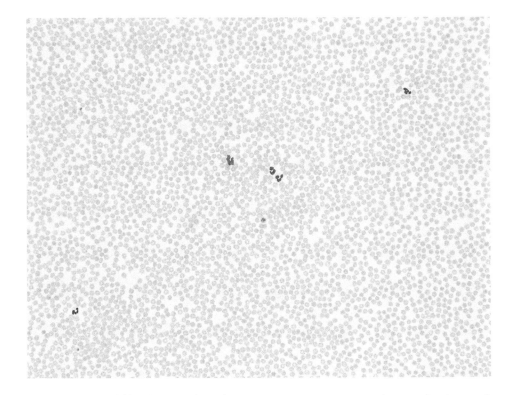

Figure 65.1 Blood film showing thrombocytopenia, neutropenia and giant platelets at the centre of the film.

As ITP is an autoimmune condition, giving a transfusion of platelets will not correct the abnormality. Platelet transfusion is reserved for emergencies, where there is serious bleeding, or when an urgent procedure needs to be done and cannot be delayed.

Patients with ITP have low levels of platelets. With a platelet count of less than $30 \times 10^9/L$ most patients will not bleed. Younger patients who are otherwise well might even tolerate platelets of less than $20 \times 10^9/L$ with no symptoms at all.

The main treatment is immunosuppression, and the first-line therapy is usually steroids, or intravenous immunoglobulins (IVIGs). Other treatment options include anti-D immunoglobulin, rituximab or TPO agonists. Steroids are given either orally or intravenously depending on severity of bleeding. The patient is usually started on a high dose of 1 mg per kg oral prednisolone or 1 g methylprednisolone intravenously.

The dose is gradually weaned off over several weeks. The patient may be kept in hospital overnight for observations, but if she is well, she can be sent home and return the next day for a review and a blood test to ensure appropriate rise in platelet count following steroids. She must be referred to a haematologist who will ensure appropriate follow-up.

ITP can be associated with infections, usually viral, and can relapse with future infections. HIV, hepatitis B, and hepatitis C should be screened for. It can also be associated with autoimmune diseases; hence some physicians send an autoimmune screen at presentation.

 KEY POINTS

- ITP is an autoimmune bleeding disorder caused by increased platelet destruction and impaired production.
- Acute leukaemia needs to be excluded with any presentation with thrombocytopenia.
- Platelet transfusion is rarely needed, unless in emergency or to cover a procedure.
- In the short term, steroids work very well, and the platelet level rises appropriately, but long-term follow-up is needed with the haematology team.

CASE 66: FATIGUE AND WEIGHT LOSS

A previously healthy 55-year-old man presents to his GP with concerns regarding his energy levels; it has gotten so bad lately that he feels very tired while doing simple gardening. He has lost 10 kg of weight over the last 6 weeks. He has no previous history of heart or lung disease, and the only medication he takes is allopurinol for recurrent gout. His only other symptom is slight abdominal discomfort, which he is attributing to his medication.

Examination

The patient appeared breathless, but with normal examination of cardiology and the respiratory system. His abdominal examination is also normal apart from an enlarged spleen. Temperature is 37.2°C. Blood pressure is 135/75.

🔍 INVESTIGATIONS

The GP arranges an urgent blood test:

Haemoglobin	125
White cell count	65.0
Neutrophils	50.0
Lymphocytes	4.0
Platelets	430
Mean corpuscular volume	82
C-reactive protein	6

Blood film is shown in Figure 66.1.

The patient is referred to the local haematology clinic and is seen under the 2-week wait referral pathway.

? QUESTIONS

1. What is the most likely diagnosis?
2. What specific test would you request to confirm the diagnosis?
3. What is the management plan of this patient?

ANSWERS

The blood test shows high white cell count (with a significant neutrophilia) and a normal C-reactive protein level. So this is not an inflammatory response, especially given that the patient is apyrexial and has no signs of infection.

The blood film (Figure 66.1) shows neutrophilia, myelocytes (cells in the maturation stage previous to neutrophils) and some blast cells. This is likely to be chronic myeloid leukae-mia (CML), which is a myeloproliferative disorder characterised by clonal expansion of the myeloid mass in the bone marrow, which eventually displaces normal haemopoiesis. Many cases are diagnosed incidentally on a routine blood test that shows typical features shown in Figure 66.1. However, it can also present with the symptoms typical of those in this case.

The disease has several phases: the 'chronic' phase is when the most cases are diagnosed, and it represents the initial stage of the disease, which could last 2–7 years. It can then transform into the 'accelerated' phase, which can take months to years, before the final phase, which is known as 'blast transformation'. At this final phase, the overwhelming majority of cells are blast cells, either myeloid or lymphoid, which are non-functioning cells that occupy the bone marrow and have the potential to invade other tissues.

Note that the difference between the presentation of acute and chronic leukaemia is that in chronic leukaemia, all of the stages of maturation of blood cells are expanded in numbers, namely blast cells, promyelocytes, myelocytes, band cells and neutrophils. In acute leukae-mia, or blast transformation of CML, most cells are blast cells, and hence the bone marrow produces no effective blood cells, leading to bone marrow failure.

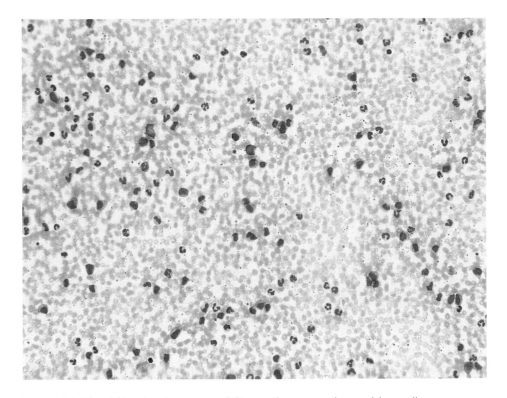

Figure 66.1 Blood film showing neutrophilia, myelocytes and some blast cells.

To confirm the diagnosis, a bone marrow biopsy to detect the *BCR-ABL1* fusion gene is needed. Some 90–95% of patients with CML have this gene, which is the result of translocation (9;22), also known as the Philadelphia chromosome.

The *ABL* gene is a proto-oncogene coding for a non-receptor tyrosine kinase. However, with the translocation of this gene onto chromosome 22, its fusion with the *BCR* produces a new oncoprotein which has a greater activity than the normal product of the *ABL* gene. The mechanism by which this new gene product affects the cell kinetics is still not fully understood.

The treatment that has changed the course of this condition is tyrosine kinase inhibitors, the first line being imatinib. This family of drugs is thought to act by binding to the oncoprotein product of the *BCR-ABL1* gene and inactivating it. Other generations of this family are available now, such as dasatinib and nilotinib.

The response to the drugs is assessed by testing three modalities: peripheral blood to ensure normalisation of blood count, cytogenetics to ensure elimination of Philadelphia-positive cells from the bone marrow and finally molecular studies to confirm the elimination of BCR-ABL1 transcript product in the circulation.

 KEY POINTS

- CML is a myeloproliferative disorder in which there is an expansion of numbers of cells at all stages of maturation.
- The condition should be suspected in any patient with persistent unexplained neutrophilia, as this might represent CML at the chronic phase.
- Tyrosine kinase inhibitors are an example of targeted therapy, in which the oncoprotein product of the *BCR-ABL1* gene is bound to and inactivated by the drug.

CASE 67: PNEUMONIA WITH ABNORMAL LIVER FUNCTION

A 32-year-old man presents to his GP with symptoms of productive cough and fever. He is not a smoker, and he does not have any past medical history. He works as a civil engineer, and he does not drink any alcohol. There is no history of any recent travel.

Examination

The patient looks unwell, his temperature is 37.9°C, and auscultation of his chest reveals crepitations in the right base. Examination of the cardiovascular and abdominal systems is unremarkable. The GP makes a diagnosis of community-acquired pneumonia and prescribes a course of amoxicillin.

The patient returns in 1 week with no improvement. The GP sends a routine blood test and a screen for atypical pneumonia, which comes back positive. He adds clarithromycin to the treatment, and the patient eventually improves.

Concerned about extrapulmonary complications of an atypical pneumonia, the GP performs a full liver screen 6 weeks later.

🔍 INVESTIGATIONS

Blood tests at the time of the pneumonia:

Haemoglobin	138
White cell count	20.0
Neutrophils	15.0
Lymphocytes	4.0
Platelets	500
Mean corpuscular volume	88
Bilirubin	20
Aspartate aminotransferase	100
Alkaline phosphatase	190
C-reactive protein	40

Atypical pneumonia screen: Serology for *Legionella* pneumonia is positive.

Liver screen 6 weeks after the pneumonia:

Bilirubin	18
Aspartate aminotransferase	114
Alkaline phosphatase	196
Ferritin	1100

Negative for HIV; CMB; EBV; hepatitis A, B and C.

Iron studies:

Serum iron	30
Transferrin saturation	70%
Total iron binding capacity	40

? **QUESTIONS**

1. What is the most likely diagnosis?
2. What other tests would you order to confirm the diagnosis?
3. What is your management plan?
4. What other advice would you give the patient regarding his lifestyle and his family?

ANSWERS

The patient had abnormal liver function tests (LFTs) at the time of his diagnosis with pneumonia. Sometimes this can be attributed to the infection. However, the LFTs remained abnormal 6 weeks after, and this suggests an alternative underlying liver pathology.

The level of ferritin increases with infection or inflammation. But at such a high level and in absence of viral liver disease, iron studies are necessary to evaluate iron status. The best test for this is transferrin saturation. In view of the elevated transferrin saturation levels, iron overload is the most likely explanation, and the most common cause for this in the Western world is haemochromatosis.

Haemochromatosis is one of the most common genetic conditions found in Northern Europe. It has four types. The most common is type 1, involving mutation in the *HFE* gene, for which the homozygous state is strongly associated with iron overload. The second most common is the H63D mutation.

Approximately one in eight people are carriers of the C282Y genetic mutation of the *HFE* gene. The function of this gene is to regulate another gene, the transferrin receptor gene, and hepcidin expression. The transferrin receptors are molecules through which transferrin binds to the cell, thereby allowing iron uptake into the cell. Hepcidin is a small peptide, expressed predominately in the liver, and is involved in iron absorption and reducing iron release from macrophages.

Patients with haemochromatosis are usually asymptomatic; the disease is usually discovered on routine screening. This patient clearly was asymptomatic. The only signs of disease were persistently deranged LFTs, which prompted further investigation. The main lesson to be drawn is not to overlook abnormal LFTs, which could have been attributed to his atypical bacterial chest infection. It is important to follow up such results after patient discharge from hospital to ensure resolution once the chest infection has cleared.

Following a confirmation of the diagnosis, screen the patients for further possible complications. Increased iron absorption from the gut encourages iron deposition in tissues. Iron could accumulate in the pancreas, causing diabetes mellitus; in the pituitary gland, causing hypogonadism; in the joints, causing arthralgia and arthritis; and in the heart, causing cardiomyopathy. The clinical assessment of haemochromatosis needs to address symptoms and signs of dysfunction in all of these organs. Appropriate tests for the function of these organs may be necessary: fasting glucose, luteinising hormone (LH), follicle-stimulating hormone (FSH), prolactin, testosterone, x-rays of joints and, if indicated, echocardiogram.

Excessive iron removal by venesection needs to be started. It is usually done at the haematology day unit by the nursing staff. The patient attends regular sessions of venesection (450 mL is usually removed each time), initially weekly, until the ferritin level is below 50 µg/L. Once this is reached, the frequency of venesection will depend on regular monitoring of ferritin to keep it below the level of 50 µg /L. Some patients will need to come every 2 weeks, but eventually most patients are established on 4- to 6-weekly sessions. Venesections may be associated with symptoms of dizziness and headaches.

All patients need to be advised about their dietary intake of iron, which needs to be reduced. Also alcohol intake ought to be reduced to avoid further liver damage.

Since haemochromatosis is an inherited condition, all first-degree family members of the patients are advised to have transferrin saturation and haemochromatosis gene tests.

🔑 **KEY POINTS**

- Haemochromatosis is a common inherited condition causing excessive iron absorption.
- Patients commonly present asymptomatically with either abnormal LFTs or elevated ferritin.
- Transferrin saturation is the best test to indicate iron overload.

CASE 68: RECURRENT EPISTAXIS

A 25-year-old man presents to the emergency department with epistaxis. He has been bleed-ing for 2 hours, and it is not responding to local pressure and ice application. The doctors call an ear, nose and throat (ENT) surgeon, who upon inspection finds a bleeding vessel in the left nostril and carries out cauterisation.

After 2 weeks, the patient returns to the emergency department with further bleeding. A repeat cauterisation is carried out, and an ENT surgery outpatient follow-up is arranged for a week later. Before the date of the follow-up, he returns to the emergency department again with bleeding from the right nostril.

Examination
At the clinic review the ENT surgeon advises that cauterisation is not the best option for the patient's recurrent bleeding, and he suggests vessel embolisation by interventional radiology to prevent further bleeding in the future.

The patient is booked for the procedure and has the following pre-procedure blood tests.

INVESTIGATIONS

Haemoglobin	101
White cell count	9.0
Platelets	500
Mean corpuscular volume	75

Urea and electrolytes are unremarkable.

Clotting screen:

Prothrombin time	11
Activated partial thromboplastin time	52
Factor VIII	60% of normal level
Factor IX	Normal level

QUESTIONS

1. How would you interpret these results? What is the differential diagnosis?
2. What further tests need to be done to confirm the diagnosis?
3. What is your management plan?

ANSWERS

This is a real case of a patient where there was a significant delay in making the correct diagnosis. The patient presented with recurrent epistaxis that needed more than treatment in the emergency department. The epistaxis should have been investigated further before sending the patient home.

One important feature here is that he is bleeding from both nostrils. If this is simply a local vessel causing the bleed, then the bleeding is expected to be from one nostril only. The fact that both nostrils are involved should arouse suspicion that the patient may have a clotting disorder.

The patient's microcytic anaemia is likely to be due to iron deficiency secondary to recurrent bleeding. His slight thrombocytosis is likely to be secondary to bleeding as well.

He has a normal PT but slightly prolonged APTT, which heightens suspicion for factor VIII and factor IX abnormalities. Factor VIII and factor IX deficiencies (i.e. haemophilia) tend to present with joint bleeding and usually at an early age. The level of factor VIII in haemophilia B is usually very low. This patient has a slightly low level, which is inconsistent with haemophilia B. However, von Willebrand factor deficiency can cause moderately low levels of factor VIII.

This patient has mucosal bleeding, which makes von Willebrand disease (VWD) the most likely diagnosis. VWD is the most common inherited bleeding disorder. The VW factor is an important element in haemostasis. It is produced predominantly by the vascular endothelium and has two main functions:

- Binding to collagen at sites of vascular injury and then capturing circulating platelets to form the initial primary haemostasis plug
- Stabilising factor VIII in the circulation by protecting it from degradation, which is why it is considered a co-factor for factor VIII

VWD can be caused by either quantitative or qualitative abnormalities of the VW factor. Patients often present in their second or third decades of life or after prolonged bleeding from a minor procedure like a tooth extraction. The usual bleeding is from mucosal surfaces, bruising, epistaxis or menorrhagia.

The patient needs to have a repeat test of factor VIII and factor IX levels as a confirmation and VW screening before any intervention is carried out. The usual VW screen includes level and functional activity. VWF:Ag measures the level of the factor, and VWF:RCo measures its activity. These tests could have been done fairly quickly, and they could have spared the patient recurrent hospital attendance and unnecessary interventions.

Artery embolisation procedures should be delayed until the confirmation of the diagnosis of VWD. For any future episodes of epistaxis, anti-fibrinolytic drugs such as tranexamic acid should be tried as a first line. Tranexamic acid works by stabilising the blood clot and usually prevents further bleeding. For recurrent bleeding not responding to tranexamic acid alone, desmopressin should be used. Intravenous desmopressin usually works within 30 minutes to produce a rise in factor VIII and VW factor levels. If this fails, then intravenous VW factor concentrate needs to be given. Such products are available only in tertiary haematology referral centres, where patients with haemophilia and VWD are usually treated. Regular follow-up is needed with the haematology team, and patient education for these conditions is essential.

🔑 KEY POINTS

- Any patient presenting with recurrent bleeding needs to have a coagulation screen.
- VWD is an inherited bleeding disorder that needs to be excluded in any patient with recurrent bleeding.
- An isolated prolonged APTT needs further evaluation and discussion with the haematology team, especially if the patient is presenting with bleeding or bruising.

CASE 69: BRUISING AFTER A PNEUMONIA

A 65-year-old woman is admitted to hospital with a community-acquired pneumonia. She was initially treated by her GP with oral antibiotics, but without any improvement, so she was admitted to hospital for IV antibiotics. She had no previous medical history apart from an appendicectomy at age 17. Over the next 48 hours she showed significant improvement in her symptoms and she was ready for discharge. The doctor is preparing her discharge letter when he is called by nursing staff to review the patient, as the patient reports some concerns regarding her skin.

Examination

The FY1 doctor examines the skin and finds some bruising over the arms and forearms. He conducts further examination and discovers that the patient has significant bruising over her back and upper legs. Otherwise, she feels well.

He sends an urgent clotting screen and decides not to delay her discharge, based on her feeling well and the limited number of beds in the hospital. The patient is sent home without reviewing the blood results.

Upon arriving home, the patient's bruising got worse, and the next morning she noticed some blood in her urine.

The FY1 doctor had meant to check the blood results the next day, but didn't have a chance because of his busy morning. The patient attended the emergency department in the afternoon with extensive bruising and epistaxis. The emergency department doctors repeated her clotting screen.

🔍 INVESTIGATIONS

Clotting screen prior to discharge:

Prothrombin time	13
Activated partial thromboplastin time	90
Fibrinogen	2.3

Clotting screen after being readmitted to the emergency department with worsening bruising and epistaxis:

Prothrombin time	14
Activated partial thromboplastin time	120
Fibrinogen	2.1

VWF:Ag and VWF:RCo: Both normal

Factor VIII: 30% of normal

Factor IX: 95% of normal

❓ QUESTIONS

1. What further questions would you ask the patient?
2. How would you interpret the clotting results, and what is the most likely diagnosis?
3. What is your management plan?

DOI: 10.1201/9781003242697-72

ANSWERS

When faced with a patient with bruising, there are several issues that doctors need to be aware of:

- Any previous history of bruising, as this may well be a normal variation in the population, and some patients may bruise more easily than others. However, this can be considered a normal variation only after a careful assessment.
- Bleeding needs to be excluded, so ask the patient about any epistaxis, haematuria, menorrhagia and haemoptysis. The major medical emergency you need to be aware of is intracranial bleeding, so careful assessment of the patient for any symptoms of headache, drowsiness or limb weakness is essential.
- Another important part of history is any previous surgical intervention, including tissue biopsy or dental work, as this would give a very good idea regarding previous haemostasis functioning. This patient had in fact had an appendicectomy many years ago, and she reports no complications.

In this patient, PT and fibrinogen are within a normal range; however, the APTT is prolonged. Since PT measures the activities of factors II, V, VII and X, this screen shows that these factors also are essentially normal.

APTT measures the activities of factors VIII, IX, XI and XII. The conclusion is that this patient has some abnormalities in one of these factors, and given that factors VIII and IX are the most clinically significant, their level of activities needs to be assessed.

Von Willebrand factor (VWF) is an important co-factor for factor VIII. VWF:Ag measures the level of the factor, and VWF:RCo measures its activity. Both tests are normal in this patient.

Factor VIII is low, and in a patient with previously unreported bleeding symptoms, this is likely to be acquired haemophilia A. This disorder presents similarly to congenital haemophilia, with bleeding subcutaneously or into the muscles, but rarely into the joints. The pathology is the result of autoantibodies associated with certain conditions which are directed against factor VIII. These antibodies can be found in autoimmune conditions such as systemic lupus erythematosus (SLE), lympho-proliferative conditions, malignancy, and infections. They can also be idiopathic, without any known associations.

Stabilising the patient is the first priority: any bleeding needs to be stopped and treated promptly. Urgent FBC needs to be sent to assess haemoglobin level and the possible need for blood transfusion.

If there is significant continuous bleeding, a bypassing agent needs to be used to correct the clotting deficiency. Two options are available: (1) activated prothrombin complex concentrate factor eight inhibitor bypassing activity (FEIBA) and (2) recombinant factor VIIa. Both preparations aim to bypass the deficiency and activate the clotting cascade further down from factor VIII, to eventually convert fibrinogen into fibrin and form a clot at the site of vascular injury.

Regardless of the bleeding, once the diagnosis is confirmed, the treatment aimed at eradicating the autoantibody needs to be started. The first line is steroids, and response is usually monitored with factor VIII serial levels. If there is no response, other options are cyclophosphamide, azathioprine or rituximab.

🔑 KEY POINTS

- Any change in the patient's condition needs to be discussed with senior colleagues prior to discharge.
- Significant bruising needs to be investigated before reassuring the patient that there is nothing wrong.
- Acquired haemophilia A is a disorder of antibodies against factor VIII.
- Treatment is immune suppression, with a bypassing agent to stop any bleeding.

CASE 70: HEADACHE AND A RASH

A 34-year-old woman presents to the emergency department with a headache. She saw her GP last week, who thought her symptoms may stem from stress at work. The headache is getting worse and is not responding to analgesia. She has no vomiting, and her headache feels like a band around her head. It was not made worse by lying flat or by straining. She also complains of coryzal symptoms. She has no significant past medical history.

Examination

She has no skin rash and her observations are all normal. Respiratory and cardiovascular examinations are both normal. Gross neurological assessments, including her reflexes, are normal. She has no photophobia. The doctors arrange routine blood tests.

While waiting for the results, she develops a high temperature of 39.4°C, and the nurse reports to the doctors that the patient has noticed a skin rash.

The doctor returns to reassess the patient, and he notices that she has become slightly vaguer about her history. On examination, she has developed a small purpuric rash over both her arms.

INVESTIGATIONS

Haemoglobin	82
White cell count	20.1
Neutrophils	15.1
Lymphocytes	3.0
Platelets	17
Reticulocytes	3.1%
Mean corpuscular volume	75
Sodium	136
Potassium	4.0
Urea	5.0
Creatinine	70
Lactate dehydrogenase	1000
Haptoglobins	Undetectable
C-reactive protein	70

Blood film shows thrombocytopenia and increased red cell fragments (Figure 70.1).

? QUESTIONS

1. What is the most likely diagnosis?
2. What test would you arrange to confirm the diagnosis?
3. What is your management plan?

ANSWERS

The patient has anaemia with a high reticulocyte percentage, raised LDH and undetectable haptoglobins, which suggests haemolysis. Haptoglobins are produced by the liver, and they are usually consumed by binding to free haemoglobin in the circulation.

Thrombocytopenia is confirmed on the blood film, which also shows increased red blood cell fragments (Figure 70.1). This is suggestive of microangiopathic haemolytic anaemia (MAHA), where the red cells are destroyed intravascularly by a mechanical force.

The presence of MAHA, thrombocytopenia, and the development of purpura with neurological symptoms are all features of thrombotic thrombocytopenic purpura (TTP). The other important differential diagnosis would be haemolytic uraemic syndrome (HUS), which in its typical type is associated with diarrhoea and renal failure.

The understanding of the pathophysiology of TTP has improved following the discovery of the role of ADAMTS-13, which is the 13th member of a family of metalloproteases. The function of this protease is to regulate the size of the von Willebrand (VW) factor molecule by cleaving the ultra-large polymers of VW factor once they are released into circulation. A deficiency in ADAMTS-13 leaves high numbers of large polymers of VW factor in circulation. These polymers are prothrombotic: they adhere to vessel walls in the microcirculation of many organs and activate passing platelets, leading to widespread platelet-rich thrombi formation.

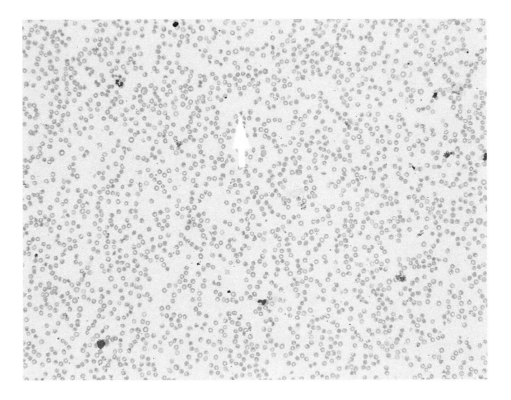

Figure 70.1 Blood film showing thrombocytopenia and increased red cell fragments.

TTP has congenital and acquired forms. The congenital form usually presents at birth and is due to an inherited deficiency of ADAMTS-13. The acquired form is secondary to either autoantibodies against ADAMTS-13, which leads to low levels of the enzyme, or massive endothelial activation releasing high numbers of the large-size VW factor molecules that exceeds the ability of the normal levels of the enzyme to regulate them.

Measurement of ADAMTS-13 serum levels would establish the diagnosis of TTP, which is a medical emergency and has a high mortality rate of 80–90%.

Plasma exchange is the treatment of choice, and it needs to be started as soon as possible. It should not be delayed until serum ADAMTS-13 results are known.

Plasma exchange is usually done at renal units or at specialist haematology units. If the hospital where the patient has presented does not have such facilities, then plasma infusion can be started until the patient is transferred. Fresh frozen plasma (FFP) should be given at a high dose; this would provide a source of functional ADAMTS-13.

 KEY POINTS

- TTP is a medical emergency which can lead to rapid deterioration of a patient.
- Deficiency in the enzyme ADAMTS-13 or widespread endothelial activation which exceeds its levels to regulate the size of VW factor polymers leads to widespread platelet activation and thrombi formation in various organs.
- Plasma exchange needs to be started promptly, and if not available, plasma infusion should be started.

CASE 71: SHORTNESS OF BREATH AND WEIGHT LOSS

A 53-year-old woman presents to her local hospital with shortness of breath. This started yesterday after she got back home from the school where she works as a dinner lady. She has not been coughing and has no pain in her chest. She has osteoarthritis in her wrists, for which she takes non-steroidal anti-inflammatory drugs (NSAIDs). She also reports some symptoms of lethargy and weight loss over the last 6 months. Occasionally she experiences sweating at night.

Examination

Her oxygen saturation is 85% on room air and 96% on 5 litres of oxygen. Her temperature is 36.5°C. She has a respiratory rate of 22 and pulse of 110. Auscultation reveals normal heart sounds and a clear chest. Her abdominal examination reveals no organomegaly. Of note, she has palpable lymph nodes in the cervical, axillary and inguinal areas.

 INVESTIGATIONS

Chest radiograph is reported as normal. The emergency department team requests a CT pulmonary angiogram (CTPA), which confirms a pulmonary embolus and enlarged anterior mediastinal, pre-tracheal, hilar, para-aortic and axillary lymph nodes.

? QUESTIONS

1. What immediate action needs to be taken based on these investigations?
2. What further investigations need to be arranged to further assess the other abnormality in the CTPA report?
3. Who else needs to get involved in the management of this patient?
4. What needs to be taken into account when treating this patient, given her initial presentation?

ANSWERS

The patient has hypoxia, tachycardia, and tachypnoea, which is a typical presentation of pulmonary embolism (PE). Based on these signs, low-molecular-weight heparin (LMWH) should be started whilst waiting for results of the investigations to confirm or exclude the PE—either CTPA or V/Q scan.

In provoked cases of PE, anticoagulation treatment should be continued for 3–6 months. Typically, it starts in the form of an LMWH, followed by oral anticoagulation. Historically, warfarin was the oral agent of choice. However, now direct oral anticoagulants (DOACs) can be used with similar effectiveness but no need for monitoring; options include rivaroxaban and apixaban. For patients started on warfarin, the target therapeutic INR is 2–3, and there needs to be a bridging period of around 48 hours when both LMWH and warfarin are used, as the onset of action of warfarin is 36–48 hours.

Many conditions are discovered as incidental findings. This patient presented with a medical emergency, but this should not distract the team from the fact that another pathology may have contributed to developing a PE.

The patient has a history of B-symptoms, including night sweats, significant weight loss (equivalent to around 10% body weight loss over 6 months) and lethargy.

In view of this history and the fact that the patient has enlarged lymph nodes, the top two differential diagnoses are lymphoma and tuberculosis (TB). Both conditions are associated with B-symptoms. However, malignancies increase the risk of developing a PE, which makes lymphoma the most likely diagnosis here. The most definitive way to confirm the diagnosis is to do a biopsy of the suspected lesion. For mediastinal lesions, cardiothoracic surgeons can perform a mediastinoscopy with a biopsy.

While waiting for the biopsy to happen, a few other investigations need to happen:

- LDH, indicating the degree of cell proliferation
- Viral screening to exclude hepatitis A, B and C and HIV infection
- Mantoux test, to screen for TB
- CT scan of chest, abdomen, and pelvis. This is called a staging CT, and its function is to exclude further lesions or lymphadenopathy. If the patient has lymph nodes in the neck, then the CT needs to include the neck in the staging

This patient should be referred to the haematology team, and the case should be discussed in the multi-disciplinary team meeting to confirm the diagnosis and decide on the management plan.

🔑 KEY POINTS

- Lymphoma can present as an incidental finding, and all suspected patients need to be screened for the presence of B-symptoms.
- Verbal reports of imaging need to be followed by formal approved reports to ensure no pathology is missed.
- Tissue biopsy is the only test that would confirm the diagnosis of a suspected lymphoma.
- Multi-disciplinary team meetings are essential in the management of patients with malignancies. Unnecessary delays usually happen in the diagnosis process because of some staging/screening tests not being done.
- Referral teams need to arrange such tests while awaiting reviews by the specialists.

CASE 72: ANAEMIA RESISTANT TO A BLOOD TRANSFUSION

A 32-year-old woman presents to the emergency department with dizziness and headaches. She had a fainting episode the day before at the school where she works as a teaching assistant. She also reports that her periods have been quite heavy lately. She has no significant past medical history, and she is not on any regular medications.

Examination

She appears pale and has a tachycardia of 120 bpm. Her BP was 80/55, and her oxygen saturation is 94%. Abdominal examination reveals splenomegaly. Examination of her heart sounds and lungs is unremarkable.

🔍 **INVESTIGATIONS**

Haemoglobin	62
White cell count	4.5
Neutrophils	2.1
Lymphocytes	2.0
Platelets	1000
Reticulocytes	6.1%
Mean corpuscular volume	110
Serum iron	20
Total iron binding capacity	50
Transferrin saturation	30%
Bilirubin	90
Aspartate aminotransferase	55
Alkaline phosphatase	100
C-reactive protein	15

Normal levels of urea and electrolytes, B_{12} and folate.

She was prescribed 2 units of packed red cells for transfusion. The following morning she had a post-transfusion blood test:

Haemoglobin	64
Mean corpuscular volume	110
White cell count	4.9
Neutrophils	2.0
Lymphocytes	2.0
Platelets	1100

❓ **QUESTIONS**

1. What is the most likely diagnosis?
2. How would you explain the post-transfusion blood results?
3. What further tests would you arrange to confirm your diagnosis?
4. What is your management plan?

DOI: 10.1201/9781003242697-75

ANSWERS

This patient has symptoms and signs consistent with anaemia. She has menorrhagia, which could cause iron-deficiency anaemia, but her pre-transfusion blood tests showed a macrocytic anaemia. Iron deficiency would cause microcytic anaemia with a low mean cell volume (MCV). This is not a combined microcytic and macrocytic anaemia, as her folate and B_{12} levels are normal.

The blood film shows polychromasia (Figure 72.1). This is a result of excessive reticulocytes, which are the cells that precede mature red cells in the maturation stages. They are larger in size, which explains the raised MCV, and are found in peripheral circulation, usually only when the bone marrow is under stress to produce more red cells. Nucleated red cells are another type of cell that are usually found only in the bone marrow, and their presence confirms that the bone marrow is under stress. The blood film shows no features of hypochromic cells typical of iron deficiency.

Bleeding, inflammation, or haemolysis may explain her thrombocytosis. The isolated raised bilirubin in addition to all of the earlier findings is supportive of haemolysis as the explanation of anaemia.

The emergency department doctor rushed to give a blood transfusion without comprehensively reviewing the results. This is a common problem in busy departments where doctors are expected to make decisions quickly. The diagnosis in this patient is haemolysis, and giving a blood transfusion to such patients would not correct the pathology. It is likely that the two units of transfusion that were given overnight were simply consumed by the haemolytic process; hence the patient's haemoglobin levels remained the same.

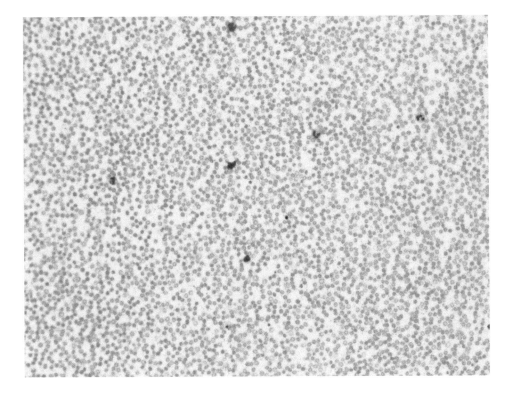

Figure 72.1 Blood film showing polychromasia, thrombocytosis and some nucleated red cells.

Haemolysis can be immune or non-immune mediated. The non-immune destruction of red cells can be mechanical, physical, chemical or associated with infections. Immune-mediated haemolysis is caused by antibodies produced against a person's own red cells (autoimmune) or towards antigens introduced to the person's body. These antigens can be introduced by drugs or via a blood transfusion (donor red cells).

The autoimmune haemolysis can be caused by antibodies active in warm temperature (warm-acting antibodies) or at cold temperatures (cold-acting antibodies). Warm autoimmune haemolytic anaemia is the most common form of immune haemolytic anaemia. The diagnosis is confirmed using the Coombs' test, also called the direct antiglobulin test (DAT). This test detects the antibodies bound to the surface of the red cells, and these antibodies can then be analysed. Haemolysis usually takes place at the spleen, hence the spleen enlargement. As the red cells coated with antibodies pass through the spleen, they are taken up and destroyed by macrophages. These cells have Fc receptors for the antibodies coating the red cells.

To confirm haemolysis, the following tests are needed:

- Blood film
- Bilirubin
- DAT
- LDH
- Haptoglobin
- Reticulocyte count

The first step in the management is to stabilise the patient. Given that she had a low blood pressure and tachycardia, fluid resuscitation has to be started as soon as possible. Once diagnosis is confirmed using the above tests, the definitive treatment for autoimmune haemolytic anaemia needs to be given in the form of immunosuppression (usually starting with high-dose steroids, which are tapered once the patient is responding).

For patients who do not respond to steroids, intravenous immunoglobulin (IVIg) should be used. IVIg is thought to work by saturating the Fc receptors of the spleen macrophages, thus preventing the uptake and destruction of red cells.

It is worth noting that warm autoimmune haemolysis can be associated with other autoimmune diseases such as systemic lupus erythematosus (SLE) or lymphoproliferative conditions such as lymphoma. Thus a careful assessment of the patient is needed to exclude other diagnoses.

🔑 KEY POINTS

- Autoimmune haemolytic anaemia can be precipitated by infections.
- Careful review of the anaemia screen helps to guide treatment and prevents unnecessary blood transfusion.
- The haemolysis screen involves blood film, bilirubin, DAT, LDH, haptoglobin and a reticulocyte count.
- Knowledge of the haemolysis screen avoids delays in the diagnosis.

CASE 73: ASYMPTOMATIC ANAEMIA IN THE ELDERLY

A 78-year-old man who is fit and well presents to his GP for an annual check-up. He only has hypertension and takes a small dose of diuretics, which keeps his blood pressure under control. His GP arranges a routine blood test.

Examination

INVESTIGATIONS

Blood test by the GP:

Haemoglobin	131	
White cell count	6.9	
Neutrophils	3.0	
Lymphocytes	2.5	
Platelets	300	
Mean corpuscular volume	85	
Bilirubin	11	
Aspartate aminotransferase	55	
Alkaline phosphatase	90	

Unremarkable levels of urea, electrolytes, calcium and phosphate.

Serum electrophoresis:

IgG 18.0	6.5 – 16.0 g/L	
IgA 1.2	0.4 – 3.5 g/L	
IgM 0.9	0.55 – 3.0 g/L	

Monoclonal band detected at IgG kappa of 18.0 g/L.

The GP subsequently makes a referral to the haematology clinic, where the patient is reviewed and is given an annual follow-up plan.

After 5 years, he has the following results:

Haemoglobin	91	
White cell count	3.0	
Neutrophils	0.7	
Lymphocytes	1.8	
Platelets	100	
Mean corpuscular volume	84	

Unremarkable levels of urea and electrolytes, calcium, phosphate and liver function tests. Serum protein electrophoresis shows an IgG kappa monoclonal band (22.0 g/L).

B_{12} and folate levels normal.

The patient is referred to the endoscopy department for a gastroscopy and colonoscopy, the results of which are normal. A whole-body MRI scan shows no lytic lesions.

? QUESTIONS

1. What is the diagnosis based on the first blood test by the GP?
2. After 5 years of follow-up, how do you explain the change in blood test results, and what is the most likely diagnosis?
3. What is the appropriate management for this patient?

ANSWERS

This patient had an IgG kappa monoclonal band detected in his initial blood test. This represents excessive production of a paraprotein by a clone of plasma cells. Excessive plasma cell proliferation causes anaemia by displacing normal bone marrow tissue, thereby affecting haemopoiesis. Excessive paraprotein production will cause interference with bone metabolism, bony lytic lesions, accumulation in the kidneys and renal failure. This patient initially had no features of end-organ damage, as his haemoglobin level, renal function and calcium level were all normal at presentation. Therefore, the patient had a monoclonal gammopathy of unknown significance (MGUS).

After 5 years, the patient developed pancytopenia (anaemia, neutropenia and thrombocytopenia), which could be a sign of end-organ damage caused by the progression of MGUS to plasma cell myeloma. However, with only a small rise in the M-band, other causes must be excluded. Progression to plasma cell myeloma would usually have a significant rise in the monoclonal band >30 g/L, more than 10% plasma cells in the bone marrow, Bence Jones proteins in the urine, and bony lytic lesions. The anaemia could also be due to blood loss, and in this age group a gastrointestinal (GI) bleed must be excluded by gastroscopy and colonoscopy.

The blood film report in this case study is crucial, as it shows low numbers of platelets and low numbers of abnormal neutrophils (Figure 73.1). These are morphological features consistent with myelodysplasia. Myelodysplastic syndromes (MDSs) are a heterogeneous group of stem cell disorders characterised by ineffective production of blood cells, dysplastic features in the bone marrow and increased risk of transforming into leukaemia. Most patients who present with MDS are over the age of 60. Approximately 15% of patients with MDS have had previous exposure to cytotoxic medications or radiotherapy.

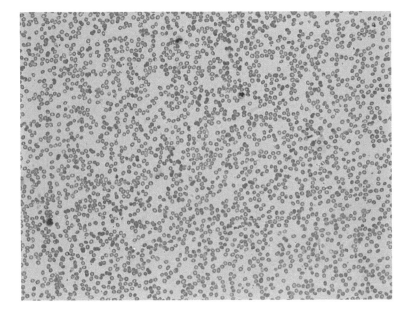

Figure 73.1 Blood film showing neutropenia, pseudo-Pelger neutrophils and hypogranulated neutrophils.

A bone marrow biopsy is needed to confirm the diagnosis of MDS and to assess the percentage of plasma cells (if <10%, then this is not progression to plasma cell myeloma). Many patients with MDS are elderly and can be managed conservatively with blood product support, and in some patients, the anaemia may respond to erythropoietin injections. This is usually done in the haematology day unit, where patients have regular blood tests to determine how often they need red cell transfusions. Usually if the haemoglobin level is below 80 g/L (or below 100 g/L in patients with a history of ischaemic heart disease), the patient will receive a red cell transfusion. Some patients may need a platelet transfusion as well to keep platelets >10.

Certain patients may qualify for chemotherapy with or without allogeneic stem cell transplantation.

In this case, the patient still has MGUS with MDS and will require follow-up for both to monitor transfusion needs and any features of progression towards plasma cell myeloma.

 KEY POINTS

- MGUS is part of the spectrum of clonal plasma cell disorders and has the risk of developing into plasma cell myeloma.
- Any changes in the patient's condition needs to be thoroughly evaluated and should not be assumed to be a progression of his disease.
- MDS is a pre-leukaemic disorder which is treated with supportive care unless the patient can tolerate chemotherapy.

CASE 74: BACK PAIN AND FATIGUE

A 55-year-old man presents to the emergency department with abdominal pain. He also reports that recently he has been getting more tired and having to take a few days off work. He has been especially complaining of back pain. He works as a manager in a food store. He has had one previous hospital admission with pneumonia. He does not take any regular medications.

Examination

He has a normal cardiovascular and respiratory examination. His abdomen is distended and slightly tender on palpation. He has no organomegaly or lymphadenopathy.

🔎 INVESTIGATIONS

Abdominal radiograph shows faecal loading but no bowel obstruction. It also shows a lytic lesion in the left pelvic bone.

His routine blood tests are:

Haemoglobin	91
White cell count	6.0
Neutrophils	4.0
Lymphocytes	2.5
Platelets	288
Mean corpuscular volume	85 fL
Sodium	141
Potassium	4.8
Urea	8.0
Creatinine	200
Bilirubin	15
Aspartate aminotransferase	52
Alkaline phosphatase	94
Calcium	3.5

Serum electrophoresis:

IgG	45.0	6.5–16.0 g/L
IgA	0.2	0.4–3.5 g/L
IgM	0.3	0.55–3.0 g/L

Monoclonal band detected an IgG kappa of 45.0 g/L.

The patient is referred to the haematology team, who perform a bone marrow biopsy, which shows excessive plasma cells with 40% infiltration of bone marrow cells.

❓ QUESTIONS

1. What is the diagnosis?
2. What further tests are needed to fully evaluate the patient?
3. What is your immediate management plan?
4. What are the possible complications of the disease?

ANSWERS

This patient has plasma cell myeloma, or multiple myeloma (MM). He has anaemia, renal failure and hypercalcaemia, the typical triad of MM.

His lethargy is secondary to either anaemia or renal failure. The abdominal pain is caused by constipation, which is secondary to high calcium levels. His back pain may well be related to lytic lesions in his spine.

MM is a condition caused by plasma cell clonal proliferation. The normal function of these cells is to produce immunoglobulins. Their production of these antibodies is normally described as polyclonal, that is, antibodies which are produced by several cells, each with its own specificity but for the same antigen. They have slightly different epitopes to match different parts of that one antigen.

In MM, there is a proliferation of one clone of plasma cells, and this proliferation produces a monoclonal protein, usually described as the M-band on the serum electrophoresis test. The excessive cell proliferation in the bone marrow disturbs the normal haemopoiesis (production of blood cells), hence the anaemia and thrombocytopenia.

The monoclonal protein accumulates in the kidney, causing renal failure, and the adhesion of plasma cells to the stromal cells in the bone marrow causes secretion of osteoclast-activating factors. It also inhibits the factors activating the osteoblast cells. This imbalance between osteoclast and osteoblast cells leads to bone weakness.

MM is usually treated with chemotherapy. For example, young and fit patients can be started on a combination of bortezomib, thalidomide, and dexamethasone followed by consolidation with autologous stem cell transplant. In less fit patients, other available combinations include melphalan and prednisolone or lenalidomide and dexamethasone.

An MM screen includes (1) serum electrophoresis to detect the monoclonal band; (2) urine sample to check for Bence Jones proteins (BJPs); (3) serum levels of beta-2 microglobulin, which is present on all nucleated cells and is used as a marker of cell proliferation and hence useful in staging MM; and (4) whole-body MRI to check for lytic lesions.

The first step in management involves correcting the hypercalcaemia and the renal failure. Hypercalcaemia can further worsen the renal failure by causing interstitial nephritis. Hydration with intravenous fluids and giving the patient intravenous bisphosphonates will help to reduce the calcium levels and correct the renal failure. His haemoglobin level is low, but he does not have cardiovascular compromise, so there is no need for a blood transfusion at this stage.

Complications of this disease include renal failure, bone disease, and anaemia. The bone disease could cause fractures, especially in the femur, or crush fractures in the vertebrae, which can be very dangerous and could cause spinal cord compression. MM could also cause recurrent infections as a result of impaired antibody production. In some cases with very high levels, the paraprotein could also interfere with the clotting proteins and cause acquired von Willebrand disease. Another common complication is the development of plasmacytoma, which is a malignant plasma cell tumour in soft tissues or in the skeleton. These may not respond to systemic therapy (chemotherapy) and may need local radiotherapy as a treatment. MM can also be associated with amyloidosis, which would involve other features, including hypertension, an enlarged tongue or peripheral neuropathy.

KEY POINTS

- In patients with anaemia and renal failure, MM must always be excluded.
- The possible complications of MM include interfering with normal haemopoiesis (anaemia), renal impairment, bone disease and fractures, recurrent infections, clotting abnormalities and development of amyloidosis.
- Cord compression secondary to vertebral crush fractures is a medical emergency that doctors need to be aware of in patients with MM.

CASE 75: SHORT OF BREATH AND UNDERWEIGHT

A 33-year-old woman presents to her GP with lethargy and dyspnoea. She has no weight loss or night sweats. She works as a sales assistant, and she has had no recent infections, and she has not travelled abroad recently. Her medical records show that she has attended previously with concerns regarding her body image, requesting help with weight loss. Her body mass index (BMI) was last recorded as 17.

Examination
She looks thin. Heart sounds are normal apart from an ejection systolic murmur. Her lungs are clear, and she has no organomegaly or lymphadenopathy.

INVESTIGATIONS

Haemoglobin	81
White cell count	1.5
Neutrophils	0.7
Lymphocytes	0.8
Platelets	67
Mean corpuscular volume	115
Sodium	141
Potassium	4.8
Urea	5.0
Creatinine	50
Bilirubin	15
Aspartate aminotransferase	52
Alkaline phosphatase	94
Thyroid function tests	Normal

QUESTIONS
1. What is the medical emergency that must be excluded?
2. What is the most likely diagnosis?
3. What tests would you perform next to confirm the diagnosis?
4. What is the treatment?

ANSWERS

In any patient presenting with lethargy and pancytopenia (low counts of all three cell lines, namely the red cells, white cells and platelets), acute leukaemia needs to be excluded. Acute myeloid leukaemia (AML) and acute lymphoid leukaemia (ALL) usually present with constitutional symptoms such as lethargy and an isolated cytopenia or pancytopenia. Normal counts may be seen in patients who are incidentally diagnosed by routine blood tests.

A blood film is usually the test of choice to exclude acute leukaemia (Figure 75.1). Initially a senior laboratory technician screens the blood film for blast cells. Then a haematologist reviews the blood film. However, morphological assessment can be challenging, so if there are any suspicious-looking cells, the blood sample can be analysed by flow cytometry to confirm the presence of blast cells.

This patient's pancytopenia is associated with a significant macrocytosis (high MCV), which may represent a high volume of immature red cells. This may be explained by acute leukaemia whereby blast cells (immature blood cells) increase the MCV, as they are larger than mature red cells. Other causes of pancytopenia with a raised MCV include cytotoxic drugs, infections such as HIV, Epstein-Barr virus, myxoedema and systemic lupus erythematosus (SLE). Macrocytosis can also be caused by thyroid abnormalities; however, the test for this patient was normal. Given the history of low BMI, dietary deficiencies also have to be ruled out.

In practice, the most common causes of macrocytic anaemia are vitamin B_{12} and folate deficiencies. Serum levels can be checked fairly quickly. This patient was eventually found to have a mixture of low vitamin B_{12} and folate deficiencies. It is a good clinical practice to check the haematinics (iron studies, vitamin B_{12} and folate) in any patient with anaemia, as patients can have multiple deficiencies.

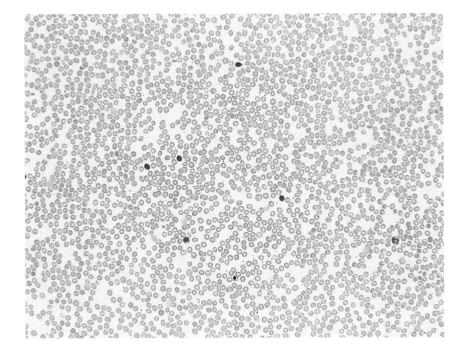

Figure 75.1 Blood film showing severe macrocytosis, with no polychromasia, neutropenia, thrombocytopenia or nucleated red blood cells seen. No blast cells are seen.

The replacement of the deficiencies should be done with care. If folate were given before vitamin B$_{12}$, the bone marrow would be stimulated to completely deplete the body of vitamin B$_{12}$ stores. This might put the patient at risk of subacute combined degeneration of the spinal cord. Hence, all such patients should have vitamin B$_{12}$ replacement first (at least one intramuscular injection) before oral folic acid is given.

Unless the patient is significantly symptomatic, she should not have a blood transfusion. Her anaemia will be corrected with vitamin B$_{12}$ and folate replacement. It is unfortunately a common mistake for clinicians to transfuse such patients. This patient is young, and her bone marrow should be healthy and able to recover once the deficiencies are corrected. She is also a women of childbearing age, so a blood transfusion would put her at risk of developing antibodies against some rare blood groups, which could affect her future pregnancies and increase the risk of her developing antibodies against her fetus's red blood cells.

The causes of the deficiencies should be further investigated. For example, further questioning is needed regarding bowel symptoms and dietary restrictions. In the case of this patient, a referral to counselling services regarding the perception of her body image and dietary intake should be considered.

 KEY POINTS

- Vitamin B$_{12}$ and folate deficiencies are common causes of macrocytic anaemia.
- Severe deficiencies can cause pancytopenia.
- Replacement with B$_{12}$ must precede folate treatment to avoid subacute combined degeneration of the spinal cord.

CASE 76: DETERIORATION AFTER A BLOOD TRANSFUSION

A 33-year-old man presents to the emergency department by ambulance, having been a victim of a major road traffic accident. During assessment, the trauma surgeon identifies an open tibial fracture from which the patient is bleeding. The patient is taken to theatre to operate on the fracture. He gives consent, and the anaesthetic team starts preparing him for the operation. He is usually fit and well, and his only significant history is a previous tonsillectomy that was complicated by excessive bleeding for which he had to receive a blood transfusion.

The patient is transfused one unit of blood. 10 minutes later the patient becomes increasingly nauseous, short of breath, sweaty, and feels dizzy. On assessment, his SpO_2 is 94% on room air, respiratory rate is 26 bpm, heart rate 110 bpm, blood pressure 95/64 mmHg, temperature 38.7°C.

INVESTIGATIONS

An urgent post-transfusion blood sample is taken:

Haemoglobin	88 g/L
Red cell count	$5.0 \times 10^{12}/L$
White cell count	$18.0 \times 10^9/L$
Platelets	$90 \times 10^9/L$
Mean corpuscular volume	87 fL

Direct antiglobulin test is positive.

Urinalysis demonstrates haemoglobinuria.

QUESTIONS

1. What do you think is the most likely explanation of the patient's deterioration?
2. Explain why the direct antiglobulin test (DAT) is positive.
3. What is your management plan?

ANSWERS

This patient had a haemolytic transfusion reaction, which is a type 2 hypersensitivity reaction that occurs within minutes to hours of exposure to a foreign red cell antigen.

Although there are more than 400 different types of antigens found on red cells, groups ABO and Rh are most likely to cause haemolytic transfusion reactions. Typically anti-A and anti-B antibodies are of the IgM class (and so associated with immediate and more severe reactions), whereas the Rh antibody (known as anti-D), which can cross the placenta during pregnancy to cause haemolytic disease of the newborn, is class IgG.

Antibodies to the ABO system are associated with complement activation and intravascular red cell lysis (haemolysis). Rh system reactions induce extravascular haemolysis within the reticuloendothelial system because Rh system antibodies cannot activate the complement cascade. Thus, phagocytes will remove IgG-coated red cells within the reticuloendothelial system. A peripheral blood smear would demonstrate small red cells, or spherocytes.

The timing and severity of the patient's deterioration, as well as the clinical sign of haemoglobinuria, indicate that an acute haemolytic transfusion reaction is taking place. This rare complication is usually caused by transfusing a patient with an incompatible red blood cell unit; this could happen through collection errors, mislabelling by the doctor or the laboratory, or mistaking a patient's identity when checking blood compatibility before the transfusion. Such a reaction can also happen if a patient has been sensitised from a previous blood transfusion. If in a blood transfusion a unit of blood containing red cell antigens is given to a patient who lacks them, antibodies against these antigens will form. If a blood unit containing the same antigens were given any time later, the patient's pre-formed antibodies would react to those antigens.

The DAT is used in cases of suspected haemolysis, while the indirect test is used in blood transfusion. DAT is simply a test to check for the presence of any antibodies or complement proteins on the surface of red cells. Their presence is not on its own a confirmation that haemolysis is taking place. Some patients with autoimmune conditions have a persistently positive DAT without any haemolysis. But in cases of proven haemolysis, it allows the clarification of the nature of the haemolysis.

In the case of this patient, he must have antibodies to the blood group of the newly transfused red cells from the donor sample. Hence, the new cells are coated with either antibodies or complement proteins, which gives the DAT a positive result. Further tests are needed to identify the nature of this antibody.

The blood transfusion should be immediately stopped, and a new blood sample from the patient needs to be sent to the laboratory along with the donor blood for repeated group and cross-matching compatibility testing. This is a medical emergency that requires immediate resuscitation, especially if the patient shows signs of shock. Intravenous fluids, chlorphenamine and hydrocortisone must be given immediately.

The transfusion laboratory needs to be informed of the incident, and the haematologist needs to get involved in reporting this reaction to the Serious Hazards of Transfusion (SHOT) group, which is a professionally lead scheme that collects and reports data related to transfusion reactions to enhance safety through the sharing of information.

🔑 **KEY POINTS**

- Patients receiving blood transfusion should be monitored regularly for signs of a transfusion reaction.
- Human error in identifying the patient is the most common cause of transfusion-related hazards.
- Following a transfusion reaction, further tests are needed to identify the cause, and reporting the case is necessary to improve the safety of blood transfusion through learning and sharing of experiences.

CASE 77: HEADACHE AND BLURRED VISION

A 45 year-old woman presents to the emergency department with a 4-day history of headache and blurred vision. She denies having photophobia, fever, or rash. She is not on any regular medications and has no past medical history. She recalls that the symptoms started 5 days after she received her second dose of the COVID-19 vaccination (ChAdOx1-S [recombinant] AstraZeneca vaccine).

Examination

On examination, she has no fever, and her cardiorespiratory observations are within normal limits. Her blood results are shown here.

🔍 INVESTIGATIONS

- Haemoglobin   125
- White cell count   13
- Platelets   43

❓ QUESTIONS

1. What is the differential diagnosis?
2. What further tests would you arrange?
3. What would be your next management step? Are there any special considerations in this case?

ANSWERS

With a recent history of the COVID-19 vaccination, one must consider vaccine-induced thrombosis presenting with cerebral venous sinus thrombosis (CVST). If excluded, then the headache could be a side effect from the recent vaccination or related to abnormalities in blood pressure or visual acuity.

Further investigations should include blood pressure measurement and CT venogram of the brain to exclude thrombosis. The patient's platelet count is low, which is suggestive of vaccine-induced immune thrombocytopenia and thrombosis (VITT). VITT may also be called vaccine-induced prothrombotic immune thrombocytopenia (VIPIT) or thrombotic thrombocytopenic syndrome (TTS).

If VITT is confirmed, then one should also request a coagulation screen, including Clauss fibrinogen assay, D-dimer measurement, and a blood film, to confirm true thrombocytopenia. To confirm the diagnosis, an enzyme-linked immunosorbent assay (ELISA) for platelet factor 4 antibodies is useful. To complete the assessment, a detailed assessment of vision by an optometrist is also required

In this case, the CT venogram did confirm a CVST. Given the history, this is very likely a vaccination-induced event. The rate of this complication is low. However, it did receive significant attention from the public and media during the height of the COVID-19 pandemic.

Other possible causes of thrombocytopenia with thrombosis other than VITT include antiphospholipid syndrome, cancer, heparin-induced thrombocytopenia, and thrombotic thrombocytopenic purpura (TTP).

Management would include anticoagulation. However, the challenge here is that the platelets are already low, which would increase the risk of bleeding as a complication from anticoagulation. A possible consideration would be to reduce the dose, for example, to give 50% of the treatment dose. However, for VITT, current guidelines would still recommend full-dose anticoagulation, using a non-heparin-based anticoagulation, for example, direct oral anticoagulants (DOACs), unless platelets are less than 30×10^9/L. If platelets are lower than 30×10^9/L, the following alternative anticoagulation strategies may reduce the risk of bleeding: either reduced dose of argatroban or a therapeutic dose of argatroban with platelet transfusion.

Also, if fibrinogen is low, replacement therapy with fibrinogen concentrate or cryoprecipitate to maintain a level of fibrinogen of at least 1.5 g/L should be given.

Despite this episode of thrombosis, current evidence would still support that this patient should still receive a booster dose with a messenger RNA (mRNA) vaccine, provided at least 12 weeks have elapsed from the implicated dose.

🔑 **KEY POINTS**

- VITT should be considered in the differential diagnosis in any patient presenting with a compatible history and a recent vaccination.
- When presenting with low platelets and thrombosis, it is important to exclude antiphospholipid syndrome, heparin-induced thrombocytopenia and TTP.

CASE 78: LOWER BACK PAIN

During a routine review in the clinic, a patient reports worsening of her chronic lower back pain. She is 76 years old and completed chemotherapy for multiple myeloma 6 months ago. Her past medical history includes asthma and degenerative spinal disease. Her presenting paraprotein before treatment was IgG kappa with 45 g/L. After treatment, this was only 2 g/L with normalisation of haemoglobin and creatinine levels.

Examination

On examination, she has no neurological signs. Two days before this latest consultation her blood tests were done with the results shown below.

INVESTIGATIONS

Haemoglobin	130 g/L
White cell count	6
Platelet count	180
Serum protein electrophoresis: IgG kappa	3 g/L
Creatinine	130 mcg/L

QUESTIONS

1. What is the differential diagnosis?
2. What further tests would you arrange?
3. What would be your next management step?

DOI: 10.1201/9781003242697-81

ANSWERS

The lower back pain could be secondary to the known degenerative changes, especially as the patient's haemoglobin level remains normal and her paraprotein level remains low. However, the creatinine level has increased, which is a matter of concern in a patient with multiple myeloma.

Further tests should include MRI of the lower spine and light chain analysis. In this patient the MRI scan shows a large mass of 4 × 5 cm infiltrating the cauda equina. The serum free light chains (SFLC) analysis reveals a kappa light chain level of 2000 mg/L, with lambda light chain level of 60 mg/L and a ratio of kappa:lambda of 333.

This mass is likely a plasmacytoma that is causing the worsening of back pain with abnormal production of light chains. The patient is fortunate that she does not have neurological signs or symptoms, and it is therefore important to have a high level of suspicion in patients with myeloma and back pain. Light chain production is usually balanced between kappa and lambda with normal reference ranges:

- Kappa light chains: 3.3–19.4 mg/L
- Lambda light chains: 5.7–26.3 mg/L
- Normal kappa-to-lambda ratio: 0.26–1.65

However, when the ratio is significantly abnormal—for example, kappa light chains are more than seven times the level of the lambda ones—then this represents clonal production. In the case of this patient, there has been a light chain 'escape', with the monoclonal band (IgG, which has both heavy and light chains) remaining low; however, there is significant abnormal production of light chains.

In terms of management, this patient has a medical emergency, and she needs admission to hospital with a discussion with the neurosurgical team. If no surgical intervention is indicated for her cauda equina compression, then she should be referred to the clinical oncology team for radiotherapy to the plasmacytoma to prevent further progression and damage to the spine. Whilst waiting for the above, she should be started on dexamethasone, which helps to provide some initial control of the disease. After radiotherapy, further chemotherapy will still need to be given with close monitoring of the patient and the light chain levels.

 KEY POINTS

- Lower back pain in a patient with a history of plasma cell myeloma must be carefully assessed, as it could represent a relapse of the condition.
- A stable paraprotein level does not necessarily exclude a relapse of myeloma.
- Imaging and SFLC analysis must be arranged to complete the assessment in a patient with myeloma.

Section 4
MICROBIOLOGY

CASE 79: FLU-LIKE ILLNESS AFTER FOREIGN TRAVEL

A 38-year-old man presents to his local sexual health clinic for a check-up after a one-time heterosexual encounter with a new partner while he was away on a business trip in the Far East 4 weeks ago. He does not report any genitourinary symptoms at present or in the previous weeks. On direct questioning, he recalls that he was feeling "generally unwell" last week and ascribed it to the flu. He has no active medical problems and takes no medications.

Examination
General, systemic, and urogenital examinations are unremarkable.

 INVESTIGATIONS

- FBC, U+E, LFT: Normal
- Urethral swab: Negative for gonorrhoea
- Chlamydia urine PCR: Negative
- Syphilis, hepatitis B and hepatitis C serology: Negative
- HIV p24 Ag: Positive, confirmed on second sample
- HIV serology: Negative

? QUESTIONS

1. Explain why the patient has HIV despite the absence of positive serology.
2. Discuss the pathogenesis of the immunodeficiency arising from HIV infection.
3. Describe the natural history of HIV infection. What is the difference between HIV and acquired immunodeficiency syndrome (AIDS)?
4. What further HIV-specific investigations should be performed at this stage?
5. What prophylactic measures can be taken against opportunistic infections in HIV-infected individuals?

DOI: 10.1201/9781003242697-83

ANSWERS

Human immunodeficiency virus (HIV) is a retrovirus that has infected more than 30 million people worldwide. The laboratory diagnosis of HIV can be made genomically (detection of viral nucleic acid by polymerase chain reaction [PCR]), serologically (detection of antigens or antibodies by enzyme-linked immunosorbent assay [ELISA]), or immunologically (through detection of a low CD4 cell count). Here, the presence of the capsid protein (p24) of HIV has been confirmed but no anti-HIV antibodies have been detected. This is because the serologic response to HIV infection may take a minimum of 4–8 weeks to develop (even as long as 6 months in some cases—the 'window period').

The primary target of HIV is the immune system, and the virus predominantly infects CD4 T cells (helper T cells), as well as other immune cells such as macrophages and dendritic cells. In a subversive manner, latent infection of these cells is released when the immune system is activated—inflammatory cytokines lead to activation of NFκB, which binds the promoters of various target cytokine genes as well as sequences of the HIV genome, leading to activation of proviral DNA. When new virions bud off, cell lysis is induced (up to 2 billion CD4 T cells may be killed in this way each day). Aside from the *quantitative* impact on T cells, HIV also produces *qualitative* defects in T-cell function, with reduced proliferation in response to antigenic stimulation and a general reduction in T_H1 responses, leading to a deficit in cell-mediated immunity. It should be appreciated that CD4 T cells act as a "master regulator" of the adaptive immune response (e.g., through activating B cells and antibody production), and hence the virus indirectly causes a defect in the entire immune system.

The interplay between the virus and the immune system governs the clinical course of HIV infection, and typically, there are three phases to infection:

1. Acute retroviral syndrome: This is the primary response of an immunocompetent individual to HIV and is characterised by a flu-like illness 3–6 weeks after exposure (seen in this case).
2. Middle chronic phase: The virus is latent and the immune system is largely intact. It may be asymptomatic or characterised by generalised lymphadenopathy.
3. Full-blown AIDS: In this final phase, there is a dramatic increase in the viral load with breakdown of host defences and appearance of serious opportunistic infections, secondary neoplasms, and neurologic disease ('AIDS-defining illnesses'—e.g., *Pneumocystis,* toxoplasmosis and mycobacterial infection, Kaposi's sarcoma, and primary central nervous system [CNS] lymphoma).

As the diagnosis of HIV has been confirmed, the specific antiretroviral investigations that need to be performed include obtaining a CD4 T-cell count and the HIV viral load (detection of viral RNA by real-time PCR). There is typically an inverse relationship between the two, with the latter governing the rate of decline of the former, which predicts the susceptibility of the host to opportunistic infection. Other tests required at this stage include serologic tests for toxoplasma and cytomegalovirus (CMV), a tuberculin skin test (given the potential of reactivation or infection of tuberculosis [TB] in an immunodeficient host), an ECG (for baseline purposes prior to initiating any antiretroviral therapy), and a chest radiograph (as several HIV-related infections may produce lung disease).

Certain prophylactic measures can be taken against opportunistic infections if the patient has a high susceptibility (governed by CD4 T-cell count). For example, trimethoprim-sulphamethoxazole (Septrin) can be used to prevent *Pneumocystis carinii* pneumonia (if CD4 count is <200) and toxoplasmosis (if CD4 count is <100). Similarly, azithromycin can be used as mycobacterial prophylaxis in individuals with a CD4 count of 50 or less, while prolonged anti-tuberculous treatment is merited in any HIV-positive patient with a positive tuberculin test. Patients should also receive streptococcal, influenza and hepatitis B vaccines, regardless of CD4 count.

🔑 KEY POINTS

- Antibody responses to HIV may take a few weeks to become detectable, so caution should be observed when interpreting serology in the immediate period after potential viral transmission.
- HIV mainly infects CD4 T cells, producing both qualitative and quantitative defects in their function.
- There are three phases to HIV infection, starting with an acute retroviral syndrome, moving on to a middle latent phase, and progressing to full-blown AIDS.
- Prophylaxis against opportunistic infection is used, depending on the CD4 T-cell count.

CASE 80: LEG PAIN AND FEVERS

A 72-year-old woman complains of a 3-month history of worsening pain in the left thigh. The pain started as a deep ache and has gradually worsened. She reports feeling increasingly unwell over the last month, with fatigue and fevers. She has recently returned from a trip abroad and does not recall trauma to the leg. She also suffers from hypertension and type 2 diabetes mellitus, which is controlled by oral medication and not insulin injections.

Examination

Respiratory rate 22, oxygen saturation 98%, pulse 108, blood pressure 128/72 and temperature 37.8°C.

There is swelling extending from the left knee to the upper thigh. The overlying skin is dusky brown and warm. The entire left femur is extremely tender on palpation. Hip movements are normal, but there is restriction in left knee flexion and extension. The patient has good peripheral pulses, and no foot ulcers are noted.

INVESTIGATIONS

Bloods

Haemoglobin	11.5 g/dL
White cell count	21.6×10^9/L
Platelets	340×10^9/L
Blood glucose	12 mmol/L
C-reactive protein	247 mg/L

Radiology
A plain radiograph shows periosteal reaction and thickening of the left distal femur. MRI displays intramedullary abnormality, lamellar periosteal reaction and extensive cortical thickening extending from the distal to the proximal femur. There are also areas of cortical breach (Figure 80.1).

Microbiology
Methicillin-resistant *Staphylococcus aureus* (MRSA) screen negative. Peripheral blood and bone biopsy cultures grew methicillin-sensitive *S. aureus* (MSSA) after 1 day of incubation.

? QUESTIONS

1. What is the differential diagnosis for leg pain and fevers?
2. What is the most likely diagnosis?
3. What is the pathogenesis of this disease?
4. How is it treated?
5. Is her diabetes important?

DOI: 10.1201/9781003242697-84

ANSWERS

Pain, swelling, warmth, tenderness and immobility are the five cardinal signs of acute inflammation. This, alongside the fever, suggests an infective or inflammatory cause of the leg pain. In this patient the differential diagnosis includes cellulitis, soft tissue abscess, septic arthritis of the knee, osteomyelitis, malignancy of either bone or soft tissue, severe destructive osteoarthritis, ruptured Baker's cyst and deep vein thrombosis (DVT). The recent long-distance travel history is an important risk factor for DVT.

The raised white cells and inflammatory markers (CRP) do not accurately distinguish between infective and inflammatory conditions (including malignancy). The very high white blood cell count is suggestive of an abscess.

The most likely diagnosis, suggested by the MRI, is osteomyelitis. The classic physical findings are described above, including bony tenderness and overlying skin oedema or erythema. This is supported by the blood and bone culture results.

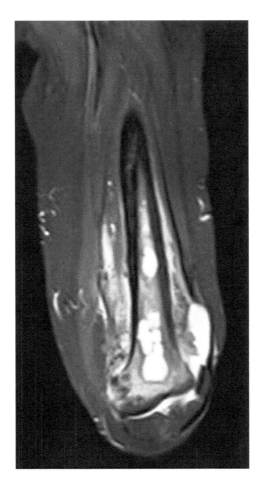

Figure 80.1 MRI of left thigh showing typical signs of osteomyelitis, including intramedullary abnormality, periosteal reaction and extensive cortical thickening extending from the distal to the proximal femur.

Osteomyelitis requires two of the following four criteria for diagnosis:

1. Pus aspirated from affected bone
2. Positive bone or blood culture
3. Positive classic localised signs
4. Positive imaging

Osteomyelitis is an infection of bone that is characterised by progressive inflammatory destruction with the formation of sequestra (dead pieces of bone within living bone), which if not treated, leads to new bone formation occurring on top of the dead and infected bone. It can affect any bone, although it occurs most commonly in the long bones.

Osteomyelitis is caused by three main pathophysiological events:

1. *Contiguous spread*: Spread from an adjacent site, which can be soft tissues or joints. More common in older adults with prosthetic joints or ulcers.
2. *Direct inoculation*: Into bone from surgery or trauma. More common in young adults.
3. *Haematogenous spread*: Spread from distant site via the bloodstream with seeding of the bone. More commonly affects long bones in children and vertebrae in adults.

The most common cause of osteomyelitis is *S. aureus*, although in osteomyelitis caused by contiguous spread from an open source (e.g., ulcer), it is often polymicrobial (caused by mixed organisms). The causative organism may be affected by patient predisposing factors. For example, Gram-negative organisms (including *Pseudomonas* spp.) are more common in diabetic patients, *Salmonella* spp. in patients with sickle cell disease and coagulase-negative staphylococci (e.g., *Staphylococcus epidermidis*) in patients with prosthetic material in their bones or joints.

Bone phagocytes engulf the bacteria and release osteolytic enzymes and toxic oxygen free radicals, which lyse the surrounding bone. Pus raises intraosseous pressure and impairs blood flow. Ischaemia results in bone necrosis and devitalised segments of bone (known as sequestra). These sequestra are important in the pathogenesis of non-resolving infection, acting as an ongoing focus of infection if not removed.

Osteomyelitis is one of the most difficult infections to treat. Treatment may require surgical debridement of necrotic tissue in addition to antibiotics, especially in chronic osteomyelitis where sequestra are present.

Antibiotic therapy is prolonged (weeks to months), and getting the microbial diagnosis is extremely important in ensuring appropriate treatment. Blood cultures will be positive in only approximately 50% of patients with osteomyelitis. Direct sampling of the bone should be attempted wherever possible in adults, particularly in chronic osteomyelitis.

Initial treatment for acute osteomyelitis is usually empiric, especially if the patient is systemically unwell and antibiotics cannot be delayed for a microbiologic diagnosis. Intravenous empirical treatment should always cover the common organisms, taking into account individual patient factors. Treatment may be changed once culture results are available.

Poorly controlled diabetics are at increased risk of infections, and having an infection leads to poor control of diabetes via altered physiology occurring during infection. Diabetics are prone to developing foot ulcers, which in turn are prone to becoming infected, which then act as a source of bacteria for infecting the contiguous bones of the feet. This process is exacerbated in patients with peripheral neuropathy, poor diabetic control, and peripheral vascular disease, as these all increase the risk of development of skin breakdown and subsequent osteomyelitis.

🔑 **KEY POINTS**

- Osteomyelitis is an infection of bone that is characterised by progressive inflammatory destruction with the formation of sequestra (dead pieces of bone within living bone). A sequestrum is caused by ischaemic necrosis to a piece of bone, causing it to die. The ischaemic necrosis is caused by raised intraosseous pressure due to pus collecting in the bone.
- The most common organism is *S. aureus*. Gram-negative bacteria, including *Pseudomonas*, affects diabetics; *Salmonella* affects patients with sickle cell disease; and staphylococci affect patients with prostheses.
- Bacteria causing osteomyelitis can be spread from adjacent sites (*contiguous spread*), from direct inoculation or from distant sites via the blood.
- Diabetes is an important risk factor where skin breakdown and ulcers can act as a source of infection.

CASE 81: FEVER AND COLLAPSE

An 80-year-old woman presents to the emergency department having been found on the floor by her daughter. She denies falling but attributed this episode to feeling increasingly unwell with fevers and malaise for the past 3 weeks. She denies any cardiorespiratory, abdominal or neurological symptoms.

Two months ago the patient had a balloon aortic valvuloplasty for severe aortic stenosis.

Examination

Oxygen saturation 86% on room air, respiratory rate 18, blood pressure 80/40, pulse 80 irregularly irregular, temperature 38.4°C.

Auscultation of the chest reveals an ejection systolic murmur loudest in the aortic region and a pansystolic murmur loudest in the mitral region. Her lung, abdomen, and neurological examination are unremarkable. A few petechial-looking lesions are found on her nail beds (as seen in Figure 81.1) and legs. Her left shoulder is warm and swollen with reduced movement in all directions.

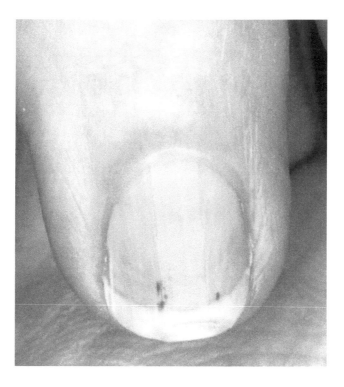

Figure 81.1 Splinter haemorrhage under fingernail.

DOI: 10.1201/9781003242697-85   243

INVESTIGATIONS

ECG was significant only for atrial fibrillation.

Bloods

Haemoglobin	11.8 g/dL
White cell count	13.0×10^9/L
Platelets	340×10^9/L
C-reactive protein	303 mg/L

Her renal function and electrolytes are unremarkable.

Radiology
Clavicular fracture
A c fracture or dislocation.
A transthoracic echocardiogram demonstrated an echogenic structure suspicious of vegetation on the anterior mitral valve leaflet.

Microbiology
Two sets of blood cultures, taken after empirical antibiotics were started, are negative to date.

QUESTIONS

1. What is the differential diagnosis of a prolonged fever?
2. What is most likely in this case?
3. What is the pathogenesis of this disease?
4. How sensitive is an echocardiogram in diagnosis?
5. What is the treatment?

ANSWERS

The differential diagnosis of a prolonged fever is broad, with main categories split into infectious (e.g., tuberculosis, Lyme disease), malignancy (e.g., lymphoma, leukaemia, or solid tumours) and inflammatory diseases (e.g., systemic lupus erythematosus [SLE], rheumatoid arthritis). Pertinent infectious causes with localising signs include infective endocarditis (IE), osteomyelitis, abscess, urinary tract infection, meningitis and cholangitis. In this case the clearly raised inflammatory markers (CRP, WBC) and high fever suggest an infectious cause is more probable. The petechiae suggest a systemic process of infection or vasculitis but may be due to trauma from a fall, although their distribution on the body makes this unlikely. There are findings on examination and investigations suggesting the source may be from the heart (endocarditis) or the shoulder. The findings of the echocardiogram make IE the most likely diagnosis.

IE is an infection of the inner lining of the heart, the endocardium. This includes the heart valves, their supporting structures, intraventricular septa and the walls of the heart, as well as any intracardiac foreign bodies, such as prosthetic valves or pacemaker wires.

Two factors are necessary for bacterial colonisation of a valve to take place:

1. Valvular damage: This can occur from turbulent blood flow, congenital heart disease, prosthetic valves, previous endocarditis, physical manipulation, the particulate material of intravenous drug user's injections and degeneration. Degenerative valves make the incidence of IE three times higher in the elderly population.
2. An inflammatory reaction to the exposed and damaged valvular endothelium results in the deposition of platelets and fibrin. Circulating bacterial colonies grow on these platelet-fibrin clots, becoming trapped in the vegetation and protected from phagocytic cells and resistant to other immune defences.

In the general population left-sided valves are predominantly affected, most often the mitral valve. Right-sided valve involvement forms less than 10% of IE and has a lower mortality than left-sided disease. Right-sided IE is more common to cohorts of intravenous drug users, congenital heart disease, and in patients with pacemakers.

The type of pathogen likely to cause IE can be determined based on factors such as the patient's age, source of infection, valve location and type (native or prosthetic) and whether the presentation is acute or subacute. Gram-positive organisms such as *Staphylococcus aureus*, *Streptococcus viridans* and enterococci are responsible for most native valve infections. Coagulase-negative staphylococci more commonly cause prosthetic valve endocarditis (PVE). *S. aureus* causes acute IE, destroying the valve quickly, with a mortality rate of 30%. This organism is typically seen on the tricuspid valve of intravenous drug users. *Staphylococcus epidermidis* commonly affects prosthetic valves within 2 months of surgery. *S. viridans* is a more low-virulence organism associated with dental procedures presenting in a subacute manner. *Streptococcus bovis* is associated with IE in those patients with colorectal carcinoma. Fungal IE can occur in immunosuppressed patients, IV drug users and prosthetic valves.

A causative organism will be identified in 90% of cases if two separate sets of blood cultures are taken 30 minutes apart. It is imperative to take blood cultures *before* antibiotics are started, which was not done in this scenario. Antibiotics are the leading cause of negative blood cultures. Another cause is intermittent shedding; therefore culture must be taken when there is a fever. Other causes of culture-negative endocarditis include the fastidious Gram-negative bacteria of the HACEK group (*Haemophilus, Aggregatibacter, Cardiobacterium, Eikenella, Kingella*),

Coxiella burnetii (Q fever) and *Bartonella* spp. Each of these three groups is responsible for up to 3% of endocarditis in England and Wales.

All patients with suspected IE must have a transthoracic echocardiogram (TTE), which detects valvular vegetations with a sensitivity of approximately 70–80%. If this is negative or there is still a high index of clinical suspicion, a transoesophageal echocardiogram (TOE) is indicated, which has a sensitivity of 90–100%. If a prosthetic valve or intracardiac device is present, a TOE is strongly recommended, as the sensitivity of the TTE is low. A follow-up echocardiogram is required at the end of antibiotic treatment to assess valve and cardiac function.

The mainstay of treatment is 4–6 weeks of high-dose IV antibiotics. About 50% of patients will require surgical intervention to remove the infected area, as host defences in heart valves are relatively ineffective. Reasons for surgical intervention are divided into three broad groups:

1. Uncontrolled infection (not responding to antibiotic therapy, a perivalvular abscess, PVE, most Gram-negative and fungal IE)
2. Prevention of embolism (very large vegetations, signs of emboli)
3. Heart failure or severe valve regurgitation

🔑 **KEY POINTS**

- IE is an infection of the inner lining of the heart, the endocardium.
- A causative organism is usually identified if blood cultures are taken before antibiotics are started.
- More than 80% of microbes responsible are Gram-positive, namely staphylococci, oral streptococci and enterococci.

CASE 82: BURNING SENSATION WHEN PASSING URINE

A 38-year-old woman presents to her GP with a 3-day history of "a burning sensation when passing urine". She reports that she voids urine more often than usual but denies a sense of urgency. She has not noticed any blood in her urine, urinary incontinence or vaginal discharge. She is sexually active and has three children, but is currently not pregnant. She also complains of severe lower back pain that started in the last day. She has never had this problem in the past and has no other medical problems. She does not take any regular medications.

Examination
Her temperature is 38.1°C. Abdominal examination reveals suprapubic tenderness but is otherwise unremarkable. There was no renal angle tenderness on either side.

 INVESTIGATIONS

Microbiology
Urinalysis is positive for nitrites, protein and leucocytes, but negative for blood. Midstream urine was collected for microscopy, culture and sensitivity. This grew *Escherichia coli* after 1 day, with sensitivity to nitrofurantoin, trimethoprim, gentamicin and co-amoxiclav. Blood cultures were not taken.

? **QUESTIONS**

1. What is the diagnosis?
2. What is the pathogenesis of this disease?
3. What are the common organisms causing this disease?
4. What complications of this disease should be excluded?
5. What is the treatment?

ANSWERS

This patient has the features of an uncomplicated urinary tract infection (UTI). Recent-onset fever and back pain suggest an upper UTI.

UTIs are classified by anatomy into lower and upper UTIs. Lower UTIs refer to infections at or below the level of the bladder and include cystitis, urethritis, prostatitis, and epididymitis (the latter three being more often sexually transmitted). Upper UTIs refer to infection above the bladder and include the ureters and kidneys. Infection of the urinary tract above the bladder is known as pyelonephritis. UTIs are also classified as complicated or uncomplicated. UTIs in men, the elderly, pregnant women, those who have an indwelling catheter and those with anatomic or functional abnormality of the urinary tract are considered to be complicated. A complicated UTI will often receive longer courses of broader-spectrum antibiotics.

Importantly, the clinical history alone of dysuria and frequency (without vaginal discharge) is associated with more than 90% probability of a UTI in healthy women.

Urine dipsticks are one of the most widely used tests, although interpreting the results is not simple. A positive result for both nitrites and leukocyte esterase has a higher sensitivity than a positive result for only one of the two. Nitrites are not normally found in the urine but are produced by the action of certain (but not all) bacteria on urinary nitrate. A positive leucocyte esterase test indicates the presence of neutrophils, a marker of infection. This infection may be a UTI, but may also be caused by other infections of the genitourinary tract. Collecting urine for microscopy, culture and sensitivity (MC&S) is the gold standard for diagnosing a UTI.

In women, a UTI develops when urinary pathogens from the bowel or vagina colonise the urethral mucosa and ascend via the urethra into the bladder. During an uncomplicated symptomatic UTI in women, it is rare for infection to ascend via the ureter into the kidney to cause pyelonephritis.

Risk factors for a UTI include being female (shorter urethra that is close to the anus), previous UTI, a urinary catheter, intercourse (which promotes movement of organisms up the urethra), use of spermicides and new sex partners.

UTI in men is uncommon and usually occurs secondary to an underlying structural or functional abnormality of the urogenital tract resulting in obstruction to urine flow. The most common of these is prostate enlargement.

Bacteria causing UTI have enhanced virulence through structures such as P fimbriae, which promote attachment to the uroepithelium. *Escherichia coli* causes 80–90% of community-acquired UTI. By contrast, only 40% of health care–associated UTIs are caused by *E. coli*. The remainder are largely due to other enteric Gram-negative bacteria such as *Klebsiella*, *Enterobacter, Serratia*, and *Pseudomonas* species. Gram-positive bacteria such as *Staphylococcus aureus* and enterococci may also cause health care–associated UTIs.

Most health care–associated UTIs are associated with the use of urinary catheters. Each day the catheter remains in situ, the risk of UTI rises by around 5%. Thus inserting catheters only when absolutely needed and ensuring they are removed as soon as possible can prevent these. In catheterised patients, the catheter becomes colonised with organisms sticking to its surface. These ascend into the bladder more easily as the urethral defences are bypassed.

Proteus species are associated with kidney stones as it produces the enzyme urease, which converts urea into ammonia, subsequently making the urine more alkaline, favouring stone development.

Complications of a UTI include:

- Recurrent cystitis in women, caused by reinfection rather than dormancy of pathogens in the uroepithelium or by ineffective treatment. There is no association between recurrent UTI and urinating habits, use of tampons, pre-coital or post-coital voiding patterns and daily fluid intake.
- Pyelonephritis, caused by bacterial migration from the bladder (via the ureters) to the kidneys. This may be life threatening or lead to permanent kidney damage if not promptly treated.
- Sepsis, which can be caused by bacteria entering the bloodstream.

Up to 40% of uncomplicated lower UTIs in women will resolve spontaneously without antimicrobial therapy. The use of antibiotics in this cohort is controversial when taking into account the side effects of antibiotics and their effect on normal flora. For this reason, a backup prescription of antibiotics can be given for uncomplicated lower UTIs to be used if symptoms get worse or do not improve in 48 hours. The antibiotics should be a short course (3 days) of a narrow spectrum, such as trimethoprim or nitrofurantoin. Resistance to trimethoprim is very high in certain areas. Complicated and upper UTIs require a longer course (e.g., 7 days) of a more broad-spectrum antibiotic such as co-amoxiclav, quinolones or aminoglycosides.

 KEY POINTS

- *E. coli* causes 80–90% of community-acquired UTI.
- Urine dipsticks are widely used, but their results must be interpreted with caution, as a significant number of false-positive and false-negative results can occur.
- An uncomplicated lower UTI is treated with a narrow-spectrum antibiotic for a short course. A complicated or upper UTI requires a longer course of a broad-spectrum antibiotic.
- Most health care–associated UTIs are associated with the use of urinary catheters. Each day the catheter remains in situ, the risk of UTI rises by around 5%.

CASE 83: A BIT SHORT OF BREATH

A 54-year-old woman presents to the emergency department with a 4-day history of worsening shortness of breath associated with pleuritic chest pain and a cough productive of purulent sputum. Her SARS-CoV-2 polymerase chain reaction (PCR) test is negative. She denies any orthopnoea or paroxysmal nocturnal dyspnoea. She is confused and disoriented in person, place, and time. She was a smoker for many years, but quit 20 years ago. She is up to date with her flu and COVID-19 vaccinations.

Examination
Her temperature is 38.4°C, respiratory rate 26, pulse 85, and blood pressure 124/54. In the right base of the chest, there is dullness to percussion, bronchial breathing and coarse early inspiratory crackles. Examination of her cardiovascular system and abdomen is unremarkable. The patient was admitted to the intensive care unit, where she was put on positive pressure ventilation.

INVESTIGATIONS

Bloods

Haemoglobin	11.0 g/dL
White cell count	18.0×10^9/L
Platelets	340×10^9/L
Urea	9.4 mmol/L
Creatinine	198 µmol/L
C-reactive protein	125 mg/L

Arterial blood gases

pH	7.5
pO_2	62.1 mmHg
pCO_2	30.6 mmHg

Radiology
Chest radiography showed consolidation in the right lung base.

Microbiology
Sputum and blood culture grew heavy growth of **Streptococcus** pneumoniae sensitive to penicillin and erythromycin.

? QUESTIONS

1. What is the differential diagnosis?
2. Which organisms cause this condition?
3. What is the pathogenesis of the cultured organism?
4. How should this condition be investigated and managed? Calculate her CURB-65 score.

ANSWERS

Dyspnoea, productive cough, fever, and raised inflammatory markers point towards a lower respiratory tract infection (LRTI). The common LRTIs presenting in the community are acute bronchitis, acute exacerbations of chronic obstructive pulmonary disease (COPD) and community-acquired pneumonia (CAP).

Acute bronchitis involves infection of the large airways, namely the tracheobronchial tree. More than 90% of the time, this is due to either upper respiratory tract viruses (rhinovirus, coronavirus) or lower respiratory tract viruses (influenza, parainfluenza, metapneumovirus, respiratory syncytial virus and adenovirus). Bacterial causes account for <10% of acute bronchitis.

Acute exacerbation of COPD occurs as a sudden worsening of COPD symptoms with increased purulence and volume of sputum.

Pneumonia is an infection of the lung tissue, including alveoli and terminal bronchioles. It can be classified anatomically into:

1. *Lobar pneumonia*: Occurs in a single lobe and is limited by the anatomic boundaries of that lobe. Usually caused by bacteria such as *S. pneumoniae* and *Klebsiella*.
2. *Broncho-pneumonia*: Patchy around the bronchi,, bilateral, often seen in a bibasal distribution. Usually *S. aureus* or *Haemophilus influenzae*.
3. *Interstitial/atypical pneumonia*: Characterised by diffuse distribution in areas surrounding alveoli. This presents with minimal sputum and a low fever—hence an atypical presentation. Caused by a variety of organisms such as *Mycoplasma*, *Chlamydia psittaci* and *Legionella*.

The incidence of CAP is higher in patients who are asplenic, immunocompromised, diabetic or alcoholic, <2 years old, or >65 years old. In the elderly population of the UK, CAP is a leading cause of death from infection.

Prior to the COVID-19 pandemic, up to 40% of all CAP was caused by *S. pneumoniae*, most commonly in winter. *H. influenzae* accounted for 10%, atypical organisms such as *Mycoplasma pneumoniae* occur in winter epidemics every 4 years (11%), and *Chlamydia pneumoniae* accounts for 13%. HIV infection or recent influenza infection predisposes patients to *Staphylococcus aureus*. Since 2020, SARS-CoV-2 has been responsible for a high proportion of viral pneumonia alongside less commonly seen influenza viruses.

S. pneumoniae (pneumococcus) is a coloniser of the upper respiratory tract, and invasion into the lower respiratory tract requires either reduced host defence or increased bacterial evasion of the host immune system. All pathogens have virulence factors encoded by genes that enhance survival in the respiratory epithelium. *Pneumococcus* has over 100 genes encoding virulence factors, the strongest of which is the polysaccharide capsule. This helps the bacterium to evade phagocytosis by inhibiting the complement cascade of the innate immune system and preventing mucosal clearance by cilia. Examples of reduced defence include immune suppression such as damage to the respiratory cilia from recent influenza or smoking, older age, and HIV.

Once in the lower respiratory tract, inflammation and damage to the mucosa lead to fluid accumulation in the alveoli, which reduces the surface available for respiration, therefore resulting in hypoxia. This alveolar fluid is what is seen on the chest radiograph as consolidation.

To establish the severity of disease, predict mortality, and guide treatment, clinical judgement and severity scoring systems have been used to good effect. In the UK, the British

Thoracic Society (BTS) recommends the use of the CURB-65 score. The score awards 1 point for each of **C**onfusion, **U**rea >7 mmol/L, **R**espiratory rate >30/min, low systolic (<90 mmHg) or diastolic (<60 mmHg) **B**lood pressure and age **65** years or older. This score stratifies patients according to increasing risk of mortality or need for hospital admission. A score of 0 is associated with 0.7% mortality, score 1 = 3.2%, score 2 = 13%, score 3 = 17%, score 4 = 41.5% and score 5 = 57%. Hospitalisation is generally required for a score of 2 or above and should be considered with a score of 1 and 0 depending on social circumstances and co-morbidities.

Microbiological identification is crucial before antibiotic treatment. For patients with moderate- or high-severity CAP (CURB-65 score of 2 or more), the BTS recommends collecting blood cultures and sputum samples for microscopy, culture and sensitivity (MC&S) and a pneumococcal urine antigen test. Blood cultures are required, as pneumococci can cause invasive disease that has a higher morbidity and mortality than pneumonia alone. Molecular testing (PCR) of respiratory samples is preferable to serological investigations for atypical pathogens and viruses. All culture samples should be collected prior to commencing antimicrobial therapy to avoid false-negative cultures.

Penicillin is the treatment of choice for a fully sensitive *S. pneumoniae* pneumonia. Macrolides or doxycycline is used in penicillin-allergic patients or if atypical pneumonia is suspected. Increasing resistance, however, has led to the need to use more broad-spectrum antibiotics such as ceftriaxone or respiratory quinolones. A pneumococcal vaccination is offered to high-risk people, including diabetics; people above 65 years old; infants; chronic heart, liver or kidney disease patients; and asplenic or immunosuppressed patients

---

🔑 KEY POINTS

- Pneumonia involves infection of the alveoli and terminal bronchioles. It can be classified as lobar or broncho-pneumonia.
- Up to 40% of all CAP is caused by *S. pneumoniae,* most commonly in winter. *S. pneumoniae* has a propensity to cause invasive disease, which has a higher mortality than pneumonia alone.
- Penicillins or macrolides are commonly used to treat pneumococcal pneumonia, depending on susceptibility of the isolate.

CASE 84: UNHAPPY CAMPER

A 27-year-old woman presents with a 2-day history of flu-like symptoms, headache, joint pains and generalised tiredness. She hadn't noticed any rash.

She lives in London and went camping in the Lake District with a group of friends 2 weeks ago. They went on extended walks in areas of long grass, and because it was hot, walking in sandals and shorts most of the time. Some of the group noticed ticks on their legs at the end of a day's walking and removed them promptly.

Examination

Temperature 39.8°C, respiratory rate 16, pulse 142 beats per minute, blood pressure 121/92.

She is found to have a bull's-eye or 'target-like' rash with clearing around the central area on her posterior upper arm, as shown in Figure 84.1. She also has some cervical lymphadenopathy. She doesn't remember removing any ticks from her arm during the trip. There are no other lesions found. Aside from joint pains, no significant pathology is found on musculoskeletal examination. She is tachycardic, but the rest of her cardiorespiratory examination is normal. She has no signs of meningitis or other nervous system involvement.

🔍 INVESTIGATIONS

Routine blood investigations are all within normal range.

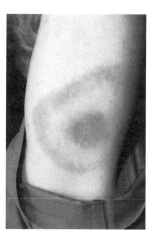

Figure 84.1 The pathognomonic erythematous rash in the pattern of a 'bull's-eye'.

❓ QUESTIONS

1. What is the most likely diagnosis?
2. What is the differential for a rash similar to Figure 84.1?
3. What are the possible complications if not treated?
4. What is the appropriate treatment?
5. How can this infection be prevented?

DOI: 10.1201/9781003242697-88

ANSWERS

Given the travel history, tick exposure, and typical rash, the most likely diagnosis is Lyme disease. Most people present 3–30 days after the bite with flu-like symptoms and a typical expanding, circular, target-like rash, which if left untreated will disappear within weeks to months. This is early, localised Lyme disease.

The typical rash, called erythema migrans, is red and expands around the site of the tick bite. Parts of the rash clear as it expands, leaving the typical 'target' or 'bull's-eye' lesion.

Other causes of similar lesions include:

- Erythema multiforme, which is caused by a cell-mediated immune reaction to drugs (antiepileptics, antibiotics, anaesthetic and non-steroidal anti-inflammatory drugs) or infections (e.g., herpes, mycoplasma). Usually presents with a generalised, blotchy, itchy rash.
- Ringworm (tinea) infection, a fungal infection occurring anywhere on the body. Its appearance is raised and scaly, and it is very itchy.
- Pityriasis rosea, a viral rash common in young women. Lesions are oval, slightly raised, mainly on the trunk and have a beige/brown colouring. They have a central clearing and are usually itchy. Rash is symmetrical on the body and often referred to as a 'fir tree' in appearance.

Lyme is the most common tick-borne infectious disease in the Northern Hemisphere, occurring in North America, Asia and Europe. It is caused by a spirochete (spiral-shaped bacterium), *Borrelia burgdorferi*, transmitted by the bite of the hard-bodied tick, *Ixodes*.

Transmission occurs during feeding when the tick injects the spirochete into the skin at the bite site. This is slow, and transmission is unlikely to occur unless the tick remains feeding for at least 36 hours. Rapid removal of ticks can prevent disease. The nymphs are tiny (poppy seed), so close inspection is needed to make sure they are removed. Most infections are due to bites by nymphs, as they are hard to see.

The spirochetes in the skin multiply, spreading outwards from the infection site. The immune reaction to the bacteria in the skin causes the typical circular rash, identifying the spreading bacteria.

Diagnosis can be based solely on typical clinical and epidemiologic criteria, including visiting a known endemic area, exposure to ticks and a typical rash. Unfortunately, not all cases give a definite history of tick exposure, and not all rashes are typical in nature. Laboratory tests may be necessary to confirm the diagnosis.

The first-line test is serological screening for antibodies against *B. burgdorferi* using enzyme-linked immunosorbent assay (ELISA). Antibodies will be produced only after exposure to the spirochete. If tested too early, the result can be negative, as it takes weeks to produce enough antibodies to be measured. If negative and there is still clinical suspicion, a second sample should be taken 2–4 weeks later and may show 'sero-conversion' from a negative to positive result, implying recent infection. The test can also be 'falsely' positive as the test cross-reacts with other infections or diseases, such as syphilis, glandular fever and rheumatoid arthritis. If the ELISA is positive, then a Western blot test should be used to confirm the diagnosis, as this test detects several antibodies to *B. burgdorferi*.

If left untreated, spirochetes will invade the bloodstream and spread to other sites. This is termed *early generalised Lyme disease* and is characterised by:

- Lyme arthritis, which usually affects the knees
- Nervous system effects, including meningitis, facial nerve palsy or other neuropathies with shooting pains
- Carditis, with abnormal heart rhythms

If still untreated or inadequately treated, this can develop into *late persistent Lyme disease* with destructive lesions and chronic, severe symptoms.

Treatment is with antibiotics, the type and duration depending on the age of the patient, presentation and severity of the disease. The antibiotics commonly used are doxycycline, amoxicillin and ceftriaxone.

Exposure to infectious agents is prevented by avoiding tick bites and wearing long socks, trousers, and long sleeves; using insect repellents; and quickly removing ticks before they are able to transmit infection. Vaccination is not available.

 KEY POINTS

- Lyme disease is the most common tick-borne infection in the Northern Hemisphere, caused by the spirochete *B. burgdorferi*.
- Clinical and epidemiologic criteria are often enough to make a diagnosis if typical. Early Lyme disease most commonly presents with flu-like symptoms and erythema migrans.
- Serology is the laboratory test of choice, but repeat tests may be needed if done too early in the infection, and confirmation of positive tests is needed to exclude false-positive reactions.
- Prevention of Lyme disease requires public awareness of avoiding tick bites and early tick removal.

CASE 85: DIARRHOEA IN AN ELDERLY MAN

An 80-year-old man living in a care home presents to the emergency department with a 4-day history of cramping abdominal pain and watery, non-bloody diarrhoea. He denies vomiting and states his diarrhoea has been worsening, with five episodes of loose stool in the past 24 hours. All of his meals are provided by the care home. No other care home residents are symptomatic. He has no recent travel history.

He is being treated for a catheter-associated urinary tract infection with co-amoxiclav by his GP. He had colon cancer, for which he had a partial colectomy 1 year ago. His medication includes aspirin and a proton pump inhibitor.

Examination

Temperature 38.1°C, oxygen saturation 95%, respiratory rate 18, pulse 112, blood pressure 100/65 mmHg.

He has signs of mild dehydration. His abdomen is mildly distended and tender, but there are no signs of guarding or rebound tenderness. Bowel sounds are active. There is no organomegaly. His urinary catheter is draining straw-coloured urine. Rectal examination reveals a large prostate and diarrhoeal stool with no evidence of blood.

INVESTIGATIONS

Bloods

			Reference values
Haemoglobin	11.4 g/dL		11.4–15.0 g/dL
White cell count	28.5×10^9/L		3.9–10.6 g/dL
Platelets	342×10^9/L		$150–440 \times 10^9$/L
C-reactive protein	86 mg/L		<5 mg/L

Radiology
Abdominal radiograph shows dilated and thickened loops of bowel suggestive of colitis.

Microbiology
Blood cultures were negative.
Stool was sent for testing but no results are available yet.

QUESTIONS

1. What is his most likely cause, and what is the differential diagnosis of watery diarrhoea?
2. What tests would you request on the stool sample?
3. What is the appropriate treatment?

ANSWERS

The most likely cause of this elderly gentleman's watery, non-bloody diarrhoea is *Clostridium difficile* bacterial gastroenteritis, given the very high peripheral white cell count and raised inflammatory markers (CRP) associated with the following risk factors: recent hospital admission, living in a care home, antibiotic therapy, bowel surgery and being on proton pump inhibitors. Important negative features of the history include no travel, not eating out and no illness in other care home residents.

C. difficile is an anaerobic, spore-forming bacterium that is carried in the gut of some people. It causes disease (pseudomembranous colitis) through production of toxins that damage the colonic mucosa. In severe disease it can lead to toxic megacolon, bowel perforation and death.

The differential diagnosis of watery diarrhoea includes:

- *Viral*—Enterovirus, rotavirus (usually in children), and norovirus (in which vomiting is almost always present)
- *Bacterial*—*Campylobacter* spp., *C. difficile*, *Yersinia enterocolitica*, *Salmonella* sp., *Shigella* sp. (usually bloody diarrhoea), *Vibrio cholera* (associated with contact or travel to endemic areas)
- *Parasitic*—*Giardia lamblia* (appropriate travel history required) or cryptosporidium in the immunocompromised or young children
- *Toxins* (which have the shortest incubation period after exposure)—Staphylococcal food poisoning, *Bacillus cereus* toxin or enterotoxogenic *Escherichia coli*
- *Non-infectious causes*—Alcohol excess, lactose intolerance or inflammatory bowel disease

Investigations of watery diarrhoea must include a stool sample sent for:

- Microscopy and culture and sensitivity (MC&S) for bacterial causes
- Polymerase chain reaction (PCR) testing looking for viral causes
- Ova, cysts and parasites
- *C. difficile* toxin testing, as only toxin-producing strains cause disease. Culture methods for *C. difficile* are slow and no longer used for diagnosis

Blood cultures are taken to exclude urinary sepsis and Gram-negative sepsis. The latter could indicate a perforation of the gut or leakage of bowel contents that would indicate severe colonic disease.

Treatment is centred on removing risk factors as possible and treating with antibiotics (metronidazole or vancyomycin). Choice of antibiotics depends on the severity of the disease and local hospital policy. In severe or life-threatening cases, surgical management may also be required (colectomy). In chronic or recurrent cases, alternative therapy includes probiotics, faecal enemas and fidaxomicin.

Prevention is by eliminating risk factors, thereby reducing the likelihood of developing disease. Reduced transmission from person to person requires hand washing with soap and water after every contact with a patient having diarrhoea. Alcohol hand rub does not destroy the spores and is therefore not sufficient to prevent spread. All patients with *C. difficile* should be isolated because its spores are hardy and easily contaminate the environment. This is why environmental cleaning plays an important role in controlling outbreaks.

🔑 **KEY POINTS**

- Risk factors for *C. difficile* infection include being elderly, recent hospital admission, living in a care home, antibiotics, bowel surgery, laxatives, proton pump inhibitors and immune suppression.
- A stool sample must be sent for *C. difficile* toxin testing if suspected, even if the patient is not in hospital.
- Reduced transmission from person to person requires hand washing with soap and water and good environmental cleaning.
- Treatment is with an antibiotic (metronidazole or vancomycin) depending on severity of disease and local hospital policy. Removing risk factors is an important part of controlling infection.

CASE 86: A PAINFUL KNEE

A 46-year-old male presents to the emergency department complaining of a painful, swollen right knee. He has been complaining of pains in his knee for months and underwent an arthroscopy 3 weeks ago for a degenerative meniscus. He has not had any other surgery to the knee, has no prosthetic joint, and does not remember any significant trauma. He is generally fit and healthy, and he plays tennis regularly. He has no other significant medical history.

He is married and living with his wife. He denies any extramarital relations and has no history of any urethral discharge or genital ulcers. He works as a teacher and has no recent travel history.

Examination

On examination, he has an erythematous, swollen right knee. He has difficulty weight-bearing on the right leg. He had a reduced range of movement in the affected knee. His temperature was 37.5°C, blood pressure 130/80 and heart rate 90 beats/min.

🔍 INVESTIGATIONS

Bloods

Haemoglobin	13.8 g/dL
White cell count	13.0×10^9/L
Platelets	298×10^9/L
C-reactive protein	240 mg/L

Radiology
A plain radiograph of the knee shows a soft tissue swelling, but no evidence of osteomyelitis is noted.

❓ QUESTIONS

1. What is your differential diagnosis for acute monoarthritis?
2. What further investigations would you like to perform on this patient?
3. How would you manage this patient?

ANSWERS

The differential diagnosis of a unilateral swollen knee/monoarthritis includes:

1. Septic arthritis
2. Crystal-induced arthritis
   a. Gout—Uric acid crystals
   b. Pseudogout—Calcium pyrophosphate crystals
   c. Other—Calcium oxalate
3. Osteoarthritis
4. Reactive arthritis (autoimmune). Reaction to infection in another part of the body, e.g., Reiter's syndrome. Usually more than a single large joint is involved
5. Traumatic arthritis
6. Haemarthrosis—Bleeding into the knee. Occurs with minor trauma in haemophiliacs

Examination of the joint fluid is often required to aid the diagnosis. The gold standard for diagnosis of septic arthritis is joint aspiration to identify an organism. In some instances this may be difficult, and image-guided aspiration is recommended. The samples should be sent for microscopy, culture, and sensitivity; tuberculosis (TB) culture (if clinically indicated) and molecular testing (polymerase chain reaction [PCR]) if the patient has already started antibiotics. The microscopy will give an initial result of the cell count and a Gram stain. The cell count will identify whether white blood cells (indicating inflammation or infection) or red blood cells (indicating haemarthrosis) are present. The Gram stain may identify organisms present in the fluid. Polarised light microscopy is required to look for crystals. Microscopy is fairly quick and cheap. However, it is not very sensitive in identifying the pathogen (50% sensitivity). These initial results could guide empiric therapy while waiting for culture results for a more targeted therapy. In instances where antibiotics are given prior to the aspiration, organisms may be seen but will not grow on the culture media. When this occurs, molecular tests (e.g., 16s PCR) could help identify the organism.

In this patient, aspiration was performed, and the microscopy showed a high white blood cell count and Gram-positive cocci in clusters and chains. Culture results the next day grew *Staphylococcus aureus*. Microscopy for crystals was negative.

Septic arthritis is an infection of the joint space and is most often monoarticular. It carries significant morbidity to the patient and could lead to destruction of the infected joint. It can also extend into the bone, leading to osteomyelitis. Septic arthritis is most commonly due to bacterial infection, but may occasionally be caused by mycobacteria, fungi or viruses.

There are many predisposing factors for septic arthritis, and these include age, prosthetic joints, diabetes mellitus, underlying arthritis and recent procedures to the affected joint. The most common route of infection is haematogenous spread; however, direct inoculation of bacteria to the joint following procedures or trauma is also common. Septic arthritis is caused by many pathogens, the most common of which is *S. aureus*, followed by streptococci. In sexually active young adults, it is important to consider gonococcal arthritis caused by *Neisseria gonorrhoeae*. The usual presentation is that of a painful, warm, red and swollen joint, the most common site being the knee.

Treatment of septic arthritis requires appropriate surgical drainage and antibiotic therapy. Treatment with antibiotics is usually for a prolonged period. Patients are usually kept for a minimum of 2 weeks of parenteral antibiotics that are then switched to an oral option for a further 2 weeks. The duration will vary depending on the pathogen isolated and response to treatment.

Radiography is usually normal on admission. However, it must always be done to monitor changes and to have a point of comparison. Surgical drainage and washout also form part of the management to reduce the burden of infection in the joint.

🔑 KEY POINTS

- Septic arthritis is an infection of a joint, usually caused by *S. aureus* and usually monoarticular.
- Joint aspiration is the gold standard diagnostic tool for septic arthritis and identifying other causes of acute monoarthritis.
- Predisposing factors for septic arthritis include age, prosthetic joints, diabetes mellitus, underlying arthritis and recent procedures to the affected joint.
- The most common route of infection is haematogenous spread.

CASE 87: A PAIN IN THE EAR

A 55-year-old woman presents with a painful left ear, having returned from France 1 week ago, where she swam in the local river on a daily basis. Since returning, she has noticed an itch in her left ear and has regularly tried to relieve it using cotton ear buds and later eardrops from the pharmacy. This itch turned into an ache, and she noticed the cotton ear bud looked a 'dirty brown'. The ache worsened, and she now also has what feels to her like a 'blocked ear'. She has no history of headache, facial weakness, difficulty swallowing or fever.

The patient has no significant medical history.

Examination

General examination was unremarkable. She was apyrexial and had no cervical lymphadenopathy.

Examination of the left ear reveals a red and swollen external auditory canal with a yellowish crusting discharge. The auditory canal is narrowed, but the tympanic membrane is visible and looks normal. The pain is made worse by pulling on the pinna (earlobe) and pushing on the tragus of the left ear. There is no redness, swelling or tenderness on any other area of the ear or surrounding tissues.

Her voice is normal, and she has no abnormalities of her cranial nerves.

 INVESTIGATIONS

Microbiology
Swabs of the external auditory canal were sent for MC&S and fungal culture. Culture grew a mixed growth of *Pseudomonas aeruginosa* and *Staphylococcus epidermidis*. Fungal culture was negative.

? **QUESTIONS**

1. What is the clinical diagnosis?
2. What are the predisposing factors and most common cause of this condition?
3. What is the treatment?

DOI: 10.1201/9781003242697-91

ANSWERS

The diagnosis is acute otitis externa (AOE), also known as 'swimmer's ear'. AOE is distinguished from chronic otitis externa by the pathogenesis and duration of symptoms, with the former of <3 weeks duration and the latter >3 months. Otitis externa is defined as inflammation of the external auditory canal. It is similar to cellulitis of skin and soft tissue elsewhere. It is a common condition and is responsible for up to 20% of referrals to ear/nose/throat (ENT) clinics.

Most cases of acute and chronic otitis externa are caused by bacterial infection, the most common pathogen being *P. aeruginosa*. Another common bacterium is *Staphylococcus aureus*. Fungal infection such as *Candida* species and *Aspergillus niger* may be found in the chronically infected external ear canal.

This patient has a number of predisposing factors which put her at risk of developing AOE, namely regular exposure to water (swimming), trauma to the external auditory canal from foreign bodies in the ear, cotton ear buds and eardrops (especially if used after being previously opened). Eczema or other inflammatory skin conditions can predispose to chronic or recurrent infection.

Earwax protects against water and keeps the pH slightly acidic in order to inhibit bacterial growth. Removal of the wax by cleaning reduces this protective mechanism. Earphones and hearing aids can also cause trauma, increasing the risk of infection. Water exposure, alkaline eardrops and soap also act to reduce the protective acidity.

Treatment of the acute episode is with a combination of aural toilet (most commonly by using microsuction) and topical antibiotics. Systemic antibiotics are indicated only if the infection extends beyond the ear canal to surrounding structures. Topical steroids reduce inflammation and can be combined with topical antibiotics.

A severe complication of AOE is necrotising otitis externa, which is an extension of infection into the surrounding tissue and bones (osteomyelitis) at the base of the brain, with possible further extension to the cranial nerves and brain. This complication is more common in the elderly, diabetics, immunocompromised and those who have received radiotherapy to the head and neck. Treatment of this complication requires long-term systemic antibiotics and close follow-up with measurement of inflammatory markers and imaging of the skull base.

 KEY POINTS

- AOE ('swimmer's ear') is characterised by localised itching, reduced hearing and pain, especially on moving the pinna and tragus (with or without a discharge).
- The most common pathogen causing AOE is *P. aeruginosa*.
- Pathogenesis is multi-factorial and includes removal of protective earwax, trauma, and excessive moisture in the ear canal.
- Treatment of AOE is topical antibiotics, and patients should be counselled on how to prevent further episodes.

CASE 88: A RED EYE

A 27-year-old man presents with a red and painful left eye. He complains that when he wakes in the morning the eyelid of his left eye is stuck together, and he has noticed his eyelid looks a bit swollen. He says a few days ago he felt an irritation and thought he might have something in his eye, but couldn't see anything. He doesn't remember any specific trauma to the eye. He hasn't been swimming and hasn't used any eye drops recently. He has noticed a few people at work with 'pink eye' but hasn't had intimate contact with any of them. He says his vision is normal, although bright light is uncomfortable, and he hasn't noticed any redness or rash on his face other than inside his eye. He has had no urethral discharge and is in a monogamous sexual relationship. He has no significant medical history.

Examination

General examination was unremarkable. He is apyrexial, and his vital signs are normal.

As shown in Figure 88.1, his left eye is noted to be sensitive to light on examination. There is a watery discharge present. The conjunctiva is erythematous and mildly oedematous with a few small subconjunctival haemorrhages in the periphery. There is no membrane present on the conjunctiva. He has pre-auricular lymphadenopathy, but no submandibular or cervical lymph nodes are palpable.

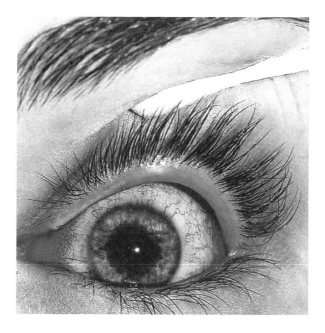

Figure 88.1 Conjuctival erythema. No ciliary injection or corenal involvement noted.

> ### ? QUESTIONS
>
> 1. What is the differential and most likely diagnosis?
> 2. What are the common organisms causing this condition?
> 3. What investigations should be done?
> 4. What is the most appropriate treatment?

DOI: 10.1201/9781003242697-92

ANSWERS

An acute red eye can be caused by many conditions, and a history and examination should guide the differential diagnosis. The following are common causes to consider:

1. Acute conjunctivitis, which can be viral, bacterial, fungal, parasitic, mycobacterial or chlamydial
2. Other eye conditions
   a. Anterior uveitis*—inflammation of the anterior structures of the uvea (the pigmented vascular inner layer of the eye comprising the iris, ciliary body and choroid)
   b. Keratitis,* i.e., corneal inflammation, which may be bacterial or viral
   c. Corneal abrasion,* foreign body,* or corneal ulcer*
   d. Acute closed-angle glaucoma*
   e. Trauma with subconjunctival haemorrhage
   f. Chemical injury*
3. Systemic conditions presenting with red eyes:
   a. Allergic conjunctivitis—Other signs of atopy should be present
   b. Measles—Commonly presenting with rash, coryza, conjunctivitis and cough
   c. Episcleritis and scleritis* associated with inflammatory bowel disease and connective tissue diseases

*These require urgent ophthalmology evaluation.

The most likely diagnosis is acute viral conjunctivitis, commonly known as 'pink eye'. It is unilateral on presentation but often spreads to infect the other eye. In its mildest form it is associated with a watery discharge, redness of the eye and eye irritation but not significant pain. If severe pain is present, other diagnoses should be sought.

The most common cause of conjunctivitis is viral, which is often associated with pre-auricular lymphadenopathy. Adenoviruses, coxsackieviruses and herpes viruses (herpes simplex virus [HSV], varicella zoster virus [VZV]) are the commonly associated viruses.

Photophobia, as in this case, suggests involvement of the cornea. A more specific diagnosis to consider is acute epidemic kerato-conjunctivitis, caused by specific strains of adenovirus. It spreads by contact or respiratory fomites and occurs most notably in schools, places of work, and institutions, where it can lead to significant outbreaks. It is more severe than other forms of adenoviral conjunctivitis and can cause marked eye pain and damage to both the conjunctiva and cornea that can lead to permanent scarring.

Bacterial conjunctivitis differs clinically in that there is usually a muco-purulent discharge and matting of the eyelids; lymphadenopathy is uncommon, and there is often an associated traumatic process predisposing to infection.

The common bacterial causes include *Staphylococcus aureus*, *Haemophilus influenzae* and *Streptococcus pneumoniae,* the latter two being more common in children than in adults. *Neisseria gonorrhoeae* causes a severe conjunctivitis and is associated with conjunctivitis in neonates born to infected mothers and sexually active adults. There is copious discharge, swelling of the conjunctiva, marked pain, and (atypically for bacterial conjunctivitis) pre-auricular lymphadenopathy. *Chlamydia trachomatis* is also associated with neonatal and sexually transmitted conjunctivitis. This causes a milder infection with less discharge and pain in the eye, but can lead to severe complications and corneal scarring with associated visual defects. In neonates it is associated with chlamydial pneumonia and therefore will require systemic as well as topical treatment.

Most cases of conjunctivitis are viral, and investigation is not necessary unless there are symptoms to suggest a more serious cause or the infection is non-resolving. If the infection is non-resolving or if a bacterial (or other non-viral) cause is suspected, appropriate swabs should be sent to the laboratory for microscopy, culture and sensitivity (MC&S) and/or molecular testing (polymerase chain reaction [PCR]) for viruses and *Chlamydia* sp., as these symptoms suggest a more serious or sight-threatening aetiology. Investigation is always indicated in neonatal conjunctivitis, as distinguishing between *C. trachomatis*, *N. gonorrhoeae* and more common bacterial causes determines treatment of the neonate and the mother and partner(s).

Most cases of viral conjunctivitis resolve spontaneously without any treatment. In more severe disease such as acute epidemic kerato-conjunctivitis, treatment is aimed at relieving symptoms and preventing spread. Patients are infectious for approximately 10–14 days after onset. If vision is affected, topical steroids may be helpful, but steroids should be prescribed only after consultation with a specialist, as these can worsen the infection. If a membrane is present, removal of this prior to the steroids may improve vision, but may lead to superficial bleeding on removal.

Bacterial and chlamydial conjunctivitis should always be treated with appropriate antibiotics. In most cases topical treatment is sufficient. The exceptions are that of neonatal *C. trachomatis*, as mentioned above, and less common causes such as chronic bacterial, fungal and parasitic infections.

Prophylaxis against neonatal conjunctivitis with topical agents is common practice, as the sequelae of untreated infection can be severe. In the UK, this has been replaced by antenatal screening, but is still commonly used in countries with a high prevalence or no resource for antenatal screening.

 KEY POINTS

- Acute viral conjunctivitis is the most common cause of inflammation of the eye. The most common organisms are adenovirus, coxsackievirus and herpes viruses.
- Red eye in patients with reduced visual acuity, photophobia, ciliary injection, corneal involvement, contact lens use or moderate pain should prompt same-day ophthalmological assessment.
- Symptoms include localised itching and irritation, redness and eye discharge.
- Treatment other than symptomatic relief is often not required, as most viral conjunctivitis resolves spontaneously. Bacterial and chlamydial conjunctivitis should always be treated with appropriate antibiotics. Corneal involvement should prompt urgent ophthalmology assessment.

CASE 89: CHILD WITH A RASH

A 3-year-old child is brought into the GP with a rash on her face, arms, legs, and body. The mother said it started on the face 4 days ago and spread to the limbs and then trunk over a few days. The child has a fever and is very irritable with poor feeding. She is up to date with her scheduled vaccinations and has been healthy since birth, which involved an uncomplicated, full-term vaginal delivery.

Examination

As shown in Figure 89.1, there is a maculopapular rash on the face, trunk, buttocks and limbs with a more extensive, symmetrical papular rash on the cheeks in a butterfly distribution. The rash on the body is coalesced in a 'lacy' pattern. There are no petechiae present. There is a mild coryza and pharyngeal erythema, but no lesions, rash or petechiae on the palate or buccal mucosa. There is no conjunctivitis present. Temperature is 37.7°C, and heart rate is 110 beats/min.

There is no lymphadenopathy or signs of meningeal irritation. The chest is clear and the abdomen soft and non-tender.

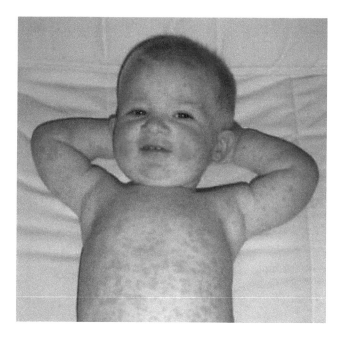

Figure 89.1 A child with a rash.

DOI: 10.1201/9781003242697-93

INVESTIGATIONS

Bloods

Haemoglobin	9.5 g/dL
Red blood cell count	$2.5 \times 10^6/mm^3$
White cell count	$9.6 \times 10^9/L$
Neutrophils	52%
Lymphocytes	45%
Platelets	$340 \times 10^9/L$
C-reactive protein	46 mg/L

? QUESTIONS

1. What is the differential diagnosis?
2. What are the pathogenesis and complications caused by the anaemia associated with infection?
3. How is the infection diagnosed?
4. What is the recommended treatment?

ANSWERS

There are a number of possible causes of childhood rashes occurring at this age. The nature of the rash and the accompanying signs and symptoms should help narrow the differential diagnosis. Historically, common childhood rashes were classified according to 'numbers', as in the table below.

Common Childhood Causes of a Maculopapular Rash with No Vesicles and No Petechiae or Purpura

Disease	Common features
Measles (first disease)	Prodrome—Coryza, cough, conjunctivitis. Rash on face, neck and shoulders. Koplik's spots on mucous membranes. Vaccine-preventable
Scarlet fever—Group A streptococcus (second disease)	Sore throat, generalised rash with perioral sparing, strawberry tongue, skin peeling following rash
Rubella (third disease)	Rapidly fading lacy rash begins on face and spreads to trunk and limbs. Suboccipital lymphadenopathy. Vaccine-preventable
Dukes' disease (fourth disease)	Unknown cause
Erythema infectiosum (fifth disease)	Slapped cheek rash, lacy rash, anaemia
Roseola infantum/exanthem subitum (sixth disease)	Pink rash beginning on trunk and spreading out to face, neck and limbs. Sore throat and red eyes
Kawasaki's disease	Need to exclude this non-infectious cause

The most likely diagnosis in this case is erythema infectiosum caused by parvovirus B19. The age of the child, typical rash and anaemia fit with this aetiology. The child is fully vaccinated, and therefore measles and rubella are unlikely causes, although there is always the slim chance of vaccine failure.

Parvovirus B19 infection results in varying manifestations depending on the presence of certain underlying conditions. Infection may be totally asymptomatic. The most common presentation is erythema infectiosum, a mild febrile illness with a rash which is more common in children aged 5–15 years old than in adults. It is commonly seen in spring months. The rash usually appears later when the viraemia has resolved and the patient is no longer infectious and can last 7–10 days. It is also known as 'slapped cheek' disease, as the facial rash appears red as if both cheeks have been slapped.

Infection is associated with an arthropathy in adults more commonly than in children, where it causes a syndrome similar to rubella with fever, rash and marked joint pain. The arthropathy is more prominent in small joints and lasts 1–3 weeks.

Parvovirus B19 is an erythrovirus, infecting red cell progenitor cells in the bone marrow, resulting in blockage of red blood cell synthesis. In healthy adults and children, this is only of minor clinical significance, and recovery of production occurs when the virus clears. This anaemia is more significant in certain groups of patients where it can lead to significant outcomes.

Complications are due mainly to the anaemia in vulnerable patient groups:

- In pregnant women, infection in the first trimester can lead to anaemia and cardiac failure in the fetus. If not treated (fetal blood transfusion), this can lead to hydrops fetalis (abnormal fluid distribution from intravascular to extravascular compartments) and death of the fetus.

- In the immunocompromised a chronic infection and chronic anaemia can occur as the immune system is not able to clear the infection. Their lack of ability to produce IgM may lead to false-negative serology tests, and this group of patients should be tested by molecular methods. Importantly, they remain infectious, as the virus is not eradicated.
- In those with underlying haematological disorders such as sickle cell disease or thalassaemia, infection can cause a transient aplastic crisis. These patients already have a reduced red cell count (due to decreased production or increased destruction), and the anaemia caused by infection pushes them into a severe aplastic crisis.

The pathogenesis of the rash and arthropathy is thought to be immune mediated through serum antibodies and immune complexes. Direct infection of the skin and synovial tissue may also contribute.

Diagnosis is usually made with a positive IgM serology for parvovirus B19. In immunocompromised patients who may not produce IgM, molecular (polymerase chain reaction [PCR]) testing looking for viral DNA is required to diagnose infection.

In healthy adults and children, no treatment is necessary, as symptoms will resolve spontaneously. In the immunocompromised, intravenous immunoglobulin (IVIG) may replace the missing immunity and assist in clearing the infection. This is not always effective, as it relies on the IVIG containing IgG to parvovirus B19. Approximately 60% of adults have had infection and therefore antibodies. In aplastic crisis a red cell transfusion may be necessary. In pregnancy intrauterine transfusion may be required to treat hydrops fetalis.

🔑 KEY POINTS

- Erythema infectiosum is a common childhood infection caused by parvovirus B19.
- The most common presentation is a mild rash, which begins on the face and spreads to the neck, trunk and extremities. The rash is often described as 'lacy' in appearance and lasts 7–10 days.
- In adults there is often an associated arthropathy lasting 1–3 weeks that makes rubella and rheumatoid arthritis common differential diagnoses.
- Treatment other than symptomatic relief is not required for healthy adults and children.
- Significant complications secondary to anaemia can occur in pregnant women, the immune compromised and those with underlying haematological disorders.

CASE 90: PELVIC PAIN

A 28-year-old teacher presents with vague lower abdominal pain. She also complains of mild pelvic discomfort on intercourse and some post-coital spotting.

She has no diarrhoea, bloating or change in bowel habits. Her menstrual cycle is normal and regular. She does not complain of vaginal discharge or itching and has no dysuria or frequency. She is sexually active and is in a monogamous relationship. She uses the oral contraceptive pill and has otherwise unprotected intercourse with her partner. She has no children and is not currently pregnant. She has no significant medical history and is otherwise fit and healthy.

Examination

She is afebrile, and her cardiorespiratory parameters are normal. There is no lymphadenopathy or jaundice present.

Her abdomen is soft with mild tenderness and guarding in the left iliac fossa. There is no rebound tenderness, and no masses can be felt. Internal pelvic examination reveals a feeling of fullness in the left iliac fossa and mild cervical motion tenderness. There is no vaginal discharge present and no blood on the glove.

INVESTIGATIONS

Radiology
Abdominopelvic ultrasound shows oedema and thickening of the left fallopian tube and free fluid in the pouch of Douglas.

Microbiology
Urine MC&S shows a high white blood cell count but no organisms and no growth. Her cervical swab tests positive for *Chlamydia trachomatis*. Both cervical and high vaginal swabs are negative for *Neisseria gonorrhoeae*.

? QUESTIONS

1. What is the diagnosis in this patient?
2. What is the pathogenesis of this disease?
3. What are the complications of this disease?
4. How is this disease treated?

ANSWERS

Her signs and symptoms are due to chlamydial infection of her fallopian tube, or salpingitis. Infection of the uterus, fallopian tubes and/or ovaries with surrounding inflammation is known collectively as pelvic inflammatory disease (PID).

Differential diagnoses of appendicitis, ectopic pregnancy, ovarian cyst, ovarian tumour, ovarian torsion, uterine fibroids, endometriosis, pyelonephritis and enteritis need to be considered.

PID is most commonly sexually transmitted and caused by *Neisseria gonorrhoeae* or *Chlamydia trachomatis*. It begins in the lower genital tract as a cervicitis or urethritis, which may be asymptomatic or present with a discharge and dysuria. If untreated, it spreads upwards to the uterus, fallopian tubes, and ovaries, causing PID. As in this patient, it can present with abnormal uterine bleeding or abdominal or pelvic pain, but is often asymptomatic and known as the 'silent disease'.

Not all PID is sexually transmitted. Other routes of infection include post-partum and post-instrumentation of the uterus or fallopian tubes, intrauterine device related and haematogenous.

Diagnosis is mainly clinical and should be considered in any sexually active woman with lower abdominal pain and genital tract tenderness on examination. Microscopy and nucleic acid amplification (NAAT) testing for *N. gonorrhoeae* and *C. trachomatis* can help to confirm the diagnosis; however, it does not exclude it. Therefore treatment should be initiated early on clinical suspicion. Testing for other sexually transmitted diseases, such as HIV and syphilis, should be considered. Current and recent sexual partners (within 6 months) should also be offered screening and treatment.

Chronic inflammation causes scarring of the reproductive organs, which can lead to infertility, ectopic pregnancies and chronic pelvic pain. A rare complication occurs when the infection spreads outside the genital tract to the peritoneum with associated scarring. If this spreads as far as the liver, it can cause a peri-hepatitis on the liver surface with adhesions to surrounding structures. This is known as Fitz-Hugh-Curtis syndrome. If a woman is pregnant with PID, this infection can cause neonatal eye and lung infections.

Treatment with antibiotics should cover both *N. gonorrhoeae* and *C. trachomatis*. Treatment should be according to the most recent guidelines and under expert advice, as resistant gonococci have emerged. Current first-line outpatient therapy according to the Centers for Disease Control and Prevention (CDC) is with 0.5 g ceftriaxone IM followed by 14 days of doxycycline. Two weeks of metronidazole can be added if there is concern of *Trichomonas* or recent vaginal instrumentation.

Prevention of PID includes the use of condoms to reduce the risk of spread. Because of its often silent nature, *Chlamydia* screening programmes have a role to play in diagnosis, reducing transmission and preventing complications.

🔑 KEY POINTS

- Infection of the uterus, fallopian tubes and/or ovaries with surrounding inflammation is known as PID.
- PID is most commonly a sexually transmitted disease caused by *N. gonorrhoeae* and *C. trachomatis*.
- PID can present with abnormal uterine bleeding or abdominal or pelvic pain, but is often silent.
- Chronic inflammation causes scarring of the reproductive organs, which can lead to infertility, ectopic pregnancies and chronic pelvic pain.
- Treatment of individual and all sexual partners is indicated, even if asymptomatic.

CASE 91: A PAINFUL, SWOLLEN JAW

A 32-year-old woman visits her dentist complaining of pain on the left side of her jaw. Over the past few weeks she has noticed increasing discomfort and some swelling in the jaw. She put it down to healing from a dental procedure until she noticed a pustule over the site of pain that has now begun to ooze a purulent fluid.

She has not lost weight and is not diabetic, immune suppressed or on any medication.

Examination

Temperature 38°C. Blood pressure and heart rate are within normal range. Her left jaw looks swollen and dark reddish in colour with a purulent liquid draining from a lesion under the angle of the jaw. The lesion feels firm and irregular to the touch. It is not painful and not obviously fluctuant. There is also a small lesion inside the mouth draining a similar purulent liquid. There is no local lymphadenopathy.

🔍 INVESTIGATIONS

Radiology
Radiograph of the jaw shows soft tissue swelling in the area of the lesion.
CT scan of the jaw shows an irregular abscess with a sinus draining externally. There is evidence of invasion of the mandible (Figure 91.1).

Microbiology
Microscopy of the drained pus reveals 'sulphur granules'. Gram stain of crushed granules shows beaded branching Gram-positive rods. Culture was negative after 24 hours.

Histopathology
Sulphur granules containing Gram-positive branching bacteria in the periphery of the granules are seen (Figure 91.2).

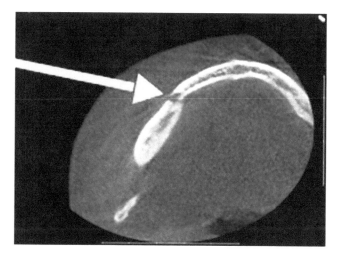

Figure 91.1 CT scan of the jaw showing mandibular destruction.

DOI: 10.1201/9781003242697-95

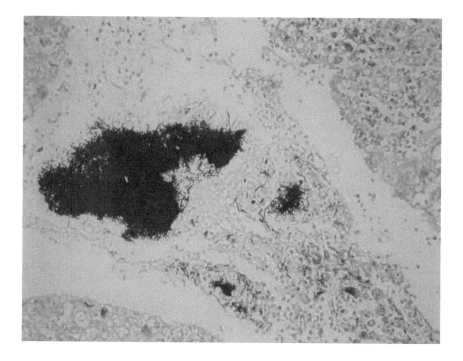

Figure 91.2 Grocott-Gomori methenamine-silver stain of a sulphur granule colony.

? QUESTIONS

1. What is the differential diagnosis?
2. How is this condition diagnosed?
3. What are the complications?
4. What is the treatment for this infection?

ANSWERS

Branching Gram-positive bacteria seen on Gram stain from a lesion on the jaw is highly suggestive of cervicofacial actinomycosis. Actinomycosis is a chronic and slowly progressive infection caused by branching, anaerobic Gram-positive bacteria of the genus *Actinomyces*, the most common species being *Actinomyces israelii*. This bacterium is normally present in the oral cavity and gastrointestinal and female genital tracts, but causes disease if it enters tissues following an injury. *A. israelii* is an anaerobic bacterium that grows very well in deep tissues where oxygen levels are low. Actinomycosis is characterised by abscesses, draining sinuses, fistulae, and tissue fibrosis. Cervicofacial actinomycosis, also known as 'lumpy jaw', is the most common presentation of this condition (50–70%) and is most often associated with dental manipulation, trauma and poor oral hygiene, the tissue damage allowing penetration of the bacteria. Other primary sites of infection include the chest, abdomen, and the pelvis in women. Central nervous system (CNS) infection, which is secondarily infected due to local or distant spread, can present with abscess formation, meningitis, meningoencephalitis or an actinomycoma. As it is usually of gradual onset, it should be considered in the diagnosis of chronic meningitis.

Actinomycosis can mimic other diseases, such that the differential diagnosis includes malignancy, fungal infection, tuberculosis (TB), lymphoma, abscesses and *Nocardia* infection (Gram-positive oral flora).

Diagnosis requires suspicion of the infection, as it is a rare condition. Clinical presentation of a chronic, indolent disease with a mass and draining sinuses, which may be recurrent or progressive, should suggest the diagnosis. Anatomically it can be cervicofacial as in the case above or, less commonly, thoracic, abdominal, pelvic or CNS. Pelvic infection in women is most often associated with the use of an intrauterine contraceptive device (IUCD).

Blood tests are non-specific and may show raised inflammatory markers. Imaging is non-specific, especially if early in the disease. CT and MRI may show an abscess or sinuses, but these are non-specific. Histopathology samples may show sulphur granules, which are colonies of organisms arranged in a mass. Gram staining of these can demonstrate Gram-positive branching bacteria. Other stains that show the bacteria are Gomori methenamine silver and Giemsa. Direct fluorescent antibody staining can be used for rapid identification.

Microbiology is the definitive diagnostic tool, as all others are non-specific. Culture of *Actinomyces* sp. from the clinical specimen is needed to confirm the diagnosis. As the organism is anaerobic, it needs to reach the lab quickly to ensure it gets cultured in the correct conditions. They are slow-growing organisms and need to be kept in culture for up to 3 weeks.

Appropriate specimens are pus, tissue and sulphur granules if visible. Swabs are not useful, as a Gram stain cannot be performed from a swab. Gram stain will reveal branching, beaded Gram-positive rods.

Newer molecular technologies such as polymerase chain reaction (PCR) and 16s rRNA sequencing may be useful if culture is negative for identifying the isolate at the species level.

Complications occur, as the diagnosis is often missed or made late in the infective process. The most common complication is extension of the infection into local structures such as surrounding muscle or bone and invasion of local soft tissue leading to fistulae and sinuses. Dissemination to distant structures is rare but can occur if left untreated.

Treatment is with antibiotics with or without surgery. Historically, prolonged (6–12 months) high-dose penicillin was used in all cases. More recently, broader-spectrum antibiotics have been used for varying periods of time depending on the site of infection, response to treatment, and species of *Actinomyces* isolated. It is best to discuss each patient with microbiology or infection specialists.

While antibiotics are the mainstay of treatment, surgery may be needed to remove infected tissue in cases that do not respond to medical treatment, when extensive sinuses or fistulae are present, when there is extensive necrosis or abscesses or when malignancy cannot be excluded.

🔑 KEY POINTS

- Actinomycosis is a chronic, slowly progressive, destructive infection caused by the anaerobic Gram-positive bacterium *Actinomyces* sp., most commonly *A. israelii*.
- Actinomycosis presents as cervicofacial (most common), thoracic, abdominal, pelvic or CNS pathology.
- Culture of *Actinomyces* sp. from the clinical specimen is needed to confirm the diagnosis, which can take up to 3 weeks.
- Treatment often involves prolonged antibiotic treatment and occasionally surgery.

CASE 92: TRAVELLER'S DIARRHOEA

A 25-year-old woman presents with a 3-week history of explosive, loose, watery diarrhoea that started 10 days after she returned from a holiday in Nepal. She drank bottled water while there, but brushed her teeth with tap water and had ice in her drinks. She opens her bowels at least five times a day and has increased flatulence. Her stools are foul smelling and float in the toilet bowl. There is no blood in the stool. The diarrhoea is associated with cramping central abdominal pain. Her appetite is unchanged, there is no vomiting, but she has noticed some weight loss. Her past medical history is unremarkable. She does not take any regular medications.

Examination

She is haemodynamically stable and not dehydrated. Her abdomen is slightly distended but is soft and non-tender to palpation. There is no organomegaly, and the liver is not tender to palpation. Auscultation reveals normal bowel sounds.

🔎 INVESTIGATIONS

Bloods
Haematology and renal and liver function tests are within normal range. Inflammatory markers are not raised.

Radiology
Abdominal x-ray showed mildly dilated loops of bowel but no evidence of obstruction.

Microbiology
No pathogens isolated from stool MC&S. Stool ova, cysts and parasites (OCP) reveal multiple cystic structures measuring 10 × 10 micrometres. These are smooth-walled and oval (Figure 92.1).

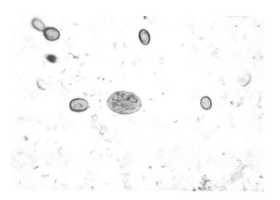

Figure 92.1 Wet mount of stool sample stained with iodine.

❓ QUESTIONS

1. What are the causes of diarrhoea in a returning traveller?
2. What is the diagnosis in this case?
3. How is this treated, and can it be prevented?

DOI: 10.1201/9781003242697-96

ANSWERS

Travellers' diarrhoea is an encompassing term of the syndrome of diarrhoea occurring in travellers. It is the most common health issue affecting returning travellers. It can be caused by a number of different organisms, including bacteria, viruses and parasites. The incubation period varies by causal agent. Onset of symptoms for viruses and bacteria range from 6 to 24 hours after exposure, whereas intestinal parasites take 1–3 weeks before the onset of symptoms. Common causes include bacteria such as *Escherichia coli* (ETEC), *Campylobacter* sp. and *Salmonella* sp., protozoa such as *Cryptosporidium* and *Giardia* spp. and viruses such as norovirus. Less common causes of diarrhoea in travellers include dysentery (*Shigella* sp.) and cholera (*Vibrio cholera*).

Travellers' diarrhoea is usually acquired through ingesting contaminated food or water. The travel destination, clinical symptom, and timing of symptoms will assist in determining the likely underlying pathogen(s). Small bowel infection usually causes watery diarrhoea, while large bowel invasion presents as dysentery (bloody diarrhoea) or colitis.

Given the chronic nature of the watery diarrhoea and the travel history in this case, the cause is more likely parasitic. The differential diagnosis would include giardiasis, or if immunocompromised, cryptosporidiosis. More than one pathogen may be associated with travellers' diarrhoea, and a full investigation for bacteria, parasites and viruses should be performed.

The patient's stool sample (Figure 92.1) contains cysts of *Giardia lamblia*. Bacterial culture is negative. This microbiological diagnosis fits with the clinical picture of watery diarrhoea, foul-smelling steatorrhea (fatty, floating stools) and abdominal cramps. *Giardia* is most prevalent in developing countries on account of poor sanitation. However, it also occurs in developed countries where water treatment is not adequate. *G. lamblia* is a protozoan parasite acquired from ingestion of cysts in contaminated water or food or by the faecal-oral route. Once in the small intestine they excyst, releasing trophozoites that bind to the small intestinal wall. Here they cause damage leading to reduced absorption of solutes, which causes an osmotic diarrhoea and malabsorption of fat and fat-soluble vitamins, resulting in steatorrhea.

Diagnosis is by stool microscopy looking for ova, cysts, and parasites. This should be requested on all patients with travellers' diarrhoea even if another pathogen is isolated, as multiple infections may occur. The cyst and trophozoite stages are both seen in the stool and will be detected in 90% of cases if stool samples are collected on 3 separate days.

Several drugs can treat giardiasis, including albendazole, tinidazole and metronidazole. The close contacts of the patient should also be screened for giardiasis.

There is no vaccine against giardiasis. Prevention of giardiasis, and other causes of travellers' diarrhoea, is best done using good food and water hygiene practices. Avoid drinking tap water or using it to brush teeth or make ice. If this is not possible, boil or treat the water before use. Drinking bottled or tinned water and drinks is preferred. Eating hot, well-cooked food and avoiding street food, undercooked food or food that has been left standing will reduce the risk. Avoid raw foods such as salads or unwashed fruits. Washing your hands before eating is essential, which can be done using soap and water or alcohol-based hand gels.

🔑 KEY POINTS

- Travellers' diarrhoea can be caused by one (or more) of a number of different organisms, including bacteria, parasites and viruses.
- *G. lamblia* is a protozoan parasite acquired from ingestion of cysts in contaminated water or food or by the faecal-oral route. *Giardia* is most prevalent in developing countries on account of poor sanitation.
- Giardiasis has a clinical picture of chronic watery diarrhoea, steatorrhea, and abdominal cramps, together with anorexia and weight loss.
- The cyst and trophozoite stages are both seen in the stool and will be detected in 90% of cases if three stool samples are collected on different days.
- Prevention of infection when travelling is best achieved through good food and water precautions.

CASE 93: FEVER IN A RETURNING TRAVELLER

A 27-year-old Ghanaian woman presents to the emergency department with a 3-day history of rigors, headache, nausea and vague lower abdominal pain. She has no significant past medical history, but is 8 weeks pregnant with her first child. She is in a monogamous relationship and denies any risky sexual contact or drug use. She lives in London and returned from a trip to Ghana 1 week ago.

She did not take malaria prophylaxis, as she is pregnant and was staying with her family in the city. She doesn't recall any bites, but was aware of the presence of mosquitoes in the environment. She ate food prepared by her mother or other family members on most occasions, although she did eat at some local take-away restaurants. She is not aware of anyone else in her household being similarly ill. She had no history of rash, joint pains, diarrhoea, jaundice, dysuria or respiratory symptoms. She does have urinary frequency that she put down to her pregnancy.

Examination

Temperature 39.8°C, blood pressure 99/60 mmHg, pulse 142 beats/min. There was no rash, no petechiae, no jaundice and no lymphadenopathy. There was no evidence of either mosquito or tick bites. Her ear/nose/throat (ENT) examination was normal.

General examination revealed some lower abdominal tenderness with some guarding. The uterus was not palpable. There is no evidence of hepatosplenomegaly or other masses in the abdomen. Respiratory and cardiovascular examinations were unremarkable aside from the tachycardia.

🔍 INVESTIGATIONS

Bloods

Haemoglobin	8.8 g/dL
White cell count	2.95×10^9/L
Platelets	41×10^9/L
Urea	8.4 mmol/L
Creatinine	178 µmol/L
Blood glucose	3.8 mmol/L
Bilirubin	72 µmol/L
Alanine aminotransferase	31 IU/L
Aspartate aminotransferase	38 IU/L
Lactate dehydrogenase	500 IU/L
C-reactive protein	82 mg/L

❓ QUESTIONS

1. Based on the clinical findings, what is your differential diagnosis?
2. Give a possible explanation of the abnormal blood results and use this together with the clinical picture to explain what additional specimens and tests you would request. What is the most likely diagnosis?
3. How may pregnancy complicate this case?
4. What is the appropriate treatment?

DOI: 10.1201/9781003242697-97

ANSWERS

Given the symptoms, signs, results and travel history, it is crucial to consider both travel-related and non-travel-related infections. In this case malaria, typhoid, hepatitis, dengue, yellow fever, schistosomiasis, SARS-CoV-2 and meningococcal disease should be considered in the differential diagnosis, as well as a urinary tract infection (UTI). Acute HIV seroconversion illness should always be considered as a differential in sexually active people.

Relevant investigations include:

- Full blood count and clotting screen, as bleeding can occur in the haemorrhagic fevers (dengue and yellow fever), meningococcal sepsis, malaria (owing to low platelets) and hepatitis (if severe liver dysfunction occurs).
- Liver function tests, as jaundice may occur in malaria, typhoid, hepatitis, dengue, yellow fever, schistosomiasis and meningococcal disease if there is severe sepsis.
- Abdominal pain and tenderness, fever, nausea, raised bilirubin and abnormal liver function tests require hepatitis studies.

Further specimens and tests suggested include:

- Urine microscopy, culture, and sensitivity (MC&S) for lower abdominal pain, fever and frequency to rule out a UTI.
- COVID-19 reverse transcription polymerase chain reaction (RT-PCR) test
- Travel plus fever requires blood cultures to exclude typhoid (abdominal pain, endemic area, fever, low platelets, low white blood cells) and meningococcal disease (endemic area, fever, low platelets).
- Abdominal pain and tenderness, anaemia and raised bilirubin require a stool sample for bacterial, viral, and parasitic pathogens.
- Travel to endemic area associated with fever, low platelets, low white blood cells and a raised LDH necessitate a malaria film. In this case microscopy of thick and thin blood smear (Figure 93.1) displays multiple ring-form trophozoites inhabiting a single, normal-sized erythrocyte, consistent with *Plasmodium falciparum* infection.
- Serum analysis for dengue was negative but is an important test because of the endemic area, fever, low platelets and low white blood cells.

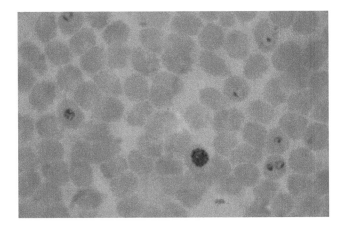

Figure 93.1 Blood smear of a *P. falciparum* culture (K1 strain). Ring stages on right and top left, including multiple rings in one red blood cell, schizont in the lower centre, trophozoite on the left.

Malaria is an acute febrile illness. In a non-immune individual, symptoms appear 7 days or more (usually 10–15 days) after the mosquito bite. The first symptoms—fever, headache, chills and vomiting—may be mild and difficult to recognise as malaria. If not treated within 24 hours, *P. falciparum* malaria can progress to severe illness often leading to death.

Worldwide malaria infects approximately 250 million and kills approximately 1 million people per year. Rising temperatures and changing weather patterns are expected to expand the burden of this disease. The majority of infection occurs in young children living in the tropics (mainly sub-Saharan Africa, Middle East, India and South America), with the most deaths occurring in sub-Saharan Africa. Five *Plasmodium* species cause malaria in humans. *P. falciparum* and *P. vivax* are the most common, with *P. falciparum* being the deadliest. The others are *P. malariae*, *P. ovale* and *P. knowlesi*. Five per cent of patients are infected with more than one species. For *P. vivax* and *P. ovale* relapses can occur weeks to months after the primary infection, as they have an inactive hypnozoite stage in the hepatocytes which can reactivate.

Transmission of the parasite occurs when the female *Anopheles* mosquito bites a human, releasing sporozoites from its salivary glands into the blood. These sporozoites enter hepatocytes where they incubate for 2–3 weeks. During this time they reproduce asexually to produce merozoites. Eventually the hepatocytes burst, releasing a mass of merozoites that rapidly invade erythrocytes, where further replication and release take place. Every 48–72 hours, the erythrocytes burst to logarithmically increase the parasite burden. Clinically, this correlates with a peak in fever every 48–72 hours, known as periodicity. This periodic fever often alternates with feeling cold and shivering. This process can result in severe anaemia.

Pathologically, erythrocytes infected with *P. falciparum* are able to adhere to and block the post-capillary blood vessels of several organs. This process can result in cerebral malaria and multi-system end-organ failure. Other complications of persistently high parasitaemia include blackwater fever (haemoglobinuria), which is a result of severe red cell destruction that produces dark urine with renal failure.

Malaria is more frequent and more complicated during pregnancy, especially in a first pregnancy. There is increased risk of maternal anaemia, respiratory complications and death from severe malaria. Miscarriage, stillbirth and intrauterine growth restriction are complications of maternal anaemia and placental infection. Prophylaxis and treatment in pregnancy are also more complicated, as some of the drugs used are contraindicated, owing to insufficient safety data or because they cause severe side effects.

Urgent treatment is necessary with expert advice. The first-line treatment of pregnant women is quinine. Hypoglycaemia, a complication of both quinine and the malarial parasite, is more common in pregnant women. Neither Coartem nor atovaquone-proguanil is recommended for use during pregnancy in the UK. Doxycycline is always contraindicated in pregnancy, and clindamycin should be used as a second drug together with quinine.

🔑 KEY POINTS

- *P. falciparum* is the most virulent species of human malaria.
- Malaria often presents with fever and non-specific symptoms and should always be considered in a traveller returning from a high-risk area.
- A thick blood film is best for screening and a thin blood film for species identification. Characteristically **P. falciparum** demonstrates a signet ring–shaped parasite surrounded by a thin cytoplasm ring. Multiple ring forms in a single erythrocyte is also characteristic.
- Malaria infection is potentially fatal and should be treated urgently with expert input.

CASE 94: A SPOT OF CONFUSION

A 16-year-old schoolboy is admitted to hospital with a 2-day history of lethargy, headache and episodes of fever and confusion. He has been physically healthy up until now. He plays football regularly and has no recent travel history. He denies any recent head trauma.

Examination

On examination he is lying under the sheets to protect his eyes from the light. His temperature is 39°C. He has marked neck stiffness. He is orientated to person and place but can't remember what day of the week it is or what he has been doing over the past few days. He has no other focal neurological signs.

He has some small, generalised lymphadenopathy. His ear/nose/throat (ENT) and respiratory tract examinations are normal. He has some small, non-blanching petechiae on his left arm and shins, which his mother has put down to his playing football. The rest of his examination is unremarkable.

INVESTIGATIONS

Bloods

Haemoglobin	13.5 g/dL
White cell count	15.4×10^9/L
Neutrophils	90%
Platelets	238×10^9/L
Blood glucose	4.6 mmol/L
C-reactive protein	144 mg/L

Imaging
A CT scan of his brain was reported as normal.

Microbiology
Blood cultures were taken after his first dose of antibiotics was given and did not grow anything.

Lumbar puncture results:

CSF results		Reference values
Protein	0.9 g/L	<0.4 g/L
Glucose	1.9 mmol/L	± 60% of blood glucose
White cell count	222	≤3 (in adult)
Neutrophils	75%	
Lymphocytes	25%	
Red cell count 128		0

Gram stain of the CSF showed Gram-negative intracellular diplococci but no growth after 5 days of incubation. TB microscopy (AFB stain) was negative.

? QUESTIONS

1. What is the differential diagnosis?
2. What other investigations would you do to confirm the suspected diagnosis?
3. What empiric antimicrobials would you start?

ANSWERS

Headache, fever, neck stiffness, photophobia and confusion suggest the diagnosis of meningitis or encephalitis. Subarachnoid haemorrhage is the most common differential but is usually more acute in onset and is associated with loss of consciousness and 'stroke-like' symptoms. Encephalitis may present like meningitis in the early stages but progresses to confusion, altered mental states, altered behaviour and speech or motor abnormalities. Subdural haematoma is unlikely in the absence of trauma. A cerebral abscess or tumour is likely to present with localising neurological signs depending on the site of the lesions. Migraine should be considered, but unless there is a past history, this is usually a diagnosis of exclusion.

Typical CSF Findings in Different Types of Meningitis

	Protein	Glucose*	Cells
Bacterial	High	Low	Very high, mainly neutrophils
Viral	Normal/high	Normal	High, mainly lymphocytes**
Tuberculosis	Very high	Low	High, mainly lymphocytes***
Cryptococcal	Normal/high	Normal/low	Few, mainly lymphocytes

*   CSF glucose normally ±60% blood glucose.
**   Can be neutrophils if herpes virus.
*** Can be neutrophils in early disease or mixed lymphocytes/neutrophils.

Common causes of meningitis are related to the age and risk factors of the patient (see table below). Underlying conditions may put them at risk of less common infections.

Age/Risk Factor		Organisms		
Neonate	Group B streptococcus	*Escherichia coli*	*Listeria monocytogenes*	
Infants and children	*Neisseria meningitidis*	*Streptococcus pneumoniae*	*Haemophilus influenzae**	
Adolescents and young adults	*S. pneumoniae*	*N. meningitidis*	Enterovirus	
Older adults	*S. pneumoniae*	*N. meningitidis*	*L. monocytogenes*	Enterovirus
All with appropriate exposure	*Mycobacterium tuberculosis*	Herpes viruses (esp. HSV-2)		
Immune suppressed	*L. monocytogenes*	*Cryptococcus neoformans*		
(In addition to those noted earlier)				
Recent neurosurgery, CSF shunts, or head trauma	*Staphylococcus aureus*	*Pseudomonas* spp.	Gram-negative bacteria	

* Reduced incidence since Hib vaccine introduced.

The clinical picture and the cerebrospinal fluid (CSF) finding of high protein, low glucose, and neutrophilic leucocytosis are most suggestive of bacterial meningitis (more specifically *Neisseria meningitidis*, a Gram-negative intracellular diplococci).

N. meningitidis is a normal inhabitant of the nasopharynx and is transmitted from person to person by secretions from the upper respiratory tract. Increased rates of meningococcal carriage occur in smokers, overcrowded households, military recruits and adolescents. Immunity is induced by carriage, and therefore established carriers do not usually develop invasive disease. The risk of invasive disease following acquisition varies with environmental, host and strain factors. The incubation period of meningococcal disease is 2–10 days. Meningitis is the most common presentation of invasive meningococcal disease and results from haematogenous dissemination of the organism.

Of the serotypes of *N. meningitidis*, six (A, B, C, W135, X and Y) are the most important clinically. Worldwide distribution of serotypes varies markedly, with type A being most prevalent in Africa and Asia but almost absent in North America and Europe, where type B is most common. Following introduction of the meningococcal C conjugate vaccination in 1999, there was a marked fall in disease caused by serogroup C strains. Since 2015, the quadrivalent vaccination (MenACWY) replaced the MenC vaccine for school children due to increasing cases of the W strain. Infants in the UK have the MenB, MenC with *Haemophilus influenza* B and pneumococcal vaccination as part of their routine immunisation schedule to prevent meningitis.

Investigations to confirm *N. meningitidis* in CSF and/or blood include:

- Blood and CSF for Gram stain and cultures and sensitivities.
- Bacterial polymerase chain reaction (PCR). A negative blood culture does not exclude a bacterial cause in this patient, as he was treated with antibiotics before blood cultures were taken. Bacterial PCR looks for bacterial DNA in the CSF or blood.
- Antigen testing of blood or CSF may provide confirmation in a patient with a clinically suspicious presentation.
- Nasopharyngeal swab looking for carriage, as this site is less affected by antibiotics than others.

Investigations looking for other pathogens are:

- Viral PCR for herpes viruses, enterovirus and adenovirus.
- Tuberculosis (TB) culture and PCR.
- Cryptococcal antigen (CRAG)—*Cryptococcus neoformans* is a fungus that commonly causes meningitis in HIV-positive patients. It usually occurs when the patient is immune suppressed with a CD4 count of below 100. This was not tested in this patient.

Treatment of meningitis is considered a medical emergency, and the first dose of antibiotics should be given within 30 minutes of presentation. Empiric treatment should cover the common causes of meningitis for the age and underlying conditions of the individual patient.

Meningococcal disease and streptococcal meningitis are both notifiable diseases, and notification must be sent to the Health Protection Agency (HPA). Close contacts (family, household, medical staff) will be assessed to determine whether prophylaxis is required. This is usually reserved for 'intimate' contacts, where there is contact with patient secretions. Patients admitted to hospital should be isolated to prevent the spread of infection.

🔑 **KEY POINTS**

- The common causes of meningitis differ in different age groups and risk groups. In healthy adults and adolescents, the most common causes are S. *pneumoniae*, *N. meningitidis* and enterovirus.
- Typical CSF findings in various forms of meningitis may be helpful in the diagnosis.
- Treatment of meningitis is an emergency, and antibiotics should be started as soon as the diagnosis is suspected.
- Meningitis is a notifiable disease.

A 28-year-old primigravid woman attends her local antenatal clinic for her routine 20-week visit. Her booking bloods taken at her 12-week visit were checked and found to be normal.

Examination
General examination was within normal limits. There was no evidence of a rash or arthritis.

 INVESTIGATIONS

Imaging
The ultrasound reveals some placental thickening, low estimated fetal weight and microcephaly.

Further History after Ultrasound Results
She works as a preschool teacher and denies any recent history of illness. On detailed questioning she admits to having a flu-like illness about 6 weeks ago. She denies having had any rash, cold sores, genital lesions, discharge or diarrhoea. She has a history of chickenpox as a child and has had her measles, mumps, rubella (MMR) vaccines. She doesn't smoke and has not drunk alcohol during her pregnancy. She doesn't have any pets at home. Her diet is healthy, and she doesn't eat any undercooked meat or unpasteurised dairy products.

? **QUESTIONS**

1. What are the causes of congenital infection, and which of these agents could cause this ultrasound result?
2. What tests can be done on the mother at this stage to determine the cause, and how would you interpret these results (see table in the Answers section)?
3. What tests can be done on the fetus at this stage to determine the cause?
4. How should this be managed during pregnancy and after delivery?

ANSWERS

Congenital infections are infections acquired in utero or during delivery. Traditionally these were known by the acronym TORCHES, representing **T**oxoplasmosis, **O**ther, **R**ubella, **C**ytomegalovirus (CMV), **HE**rpes simplex (HSV) and **S**yphilis. The 'Other' infections include varicella zoster virus (VZV), parvovirus B19, coxsackievirus and HIV.

These infections have some common presentations, but also distinctions between them, and clinical findings should be used to guide testing. In this case the pathogens likely to cause the ultrasound findings include toxoplasmosis, cytomegalovirus (CMV), herpes simplex virus (HSV) and VZV.

Maternal blood was tested for CMV, rubella, VZV, HSV and toxoplasma antibodies. Her booking bloods were compared with her current blood results:

Test	Booking blood results (12 weeks)	Current blood results (20 weeks)
Rubella IgG	+ve	+ve
Rubella IgM	−ve	−ve
VZV IgG	+ve	+ve
VZV IgM	−ve	−ve
HSV IgG	+ve	+ve
HSV IgM	−ve	−ve
CMV IgG	−ve	+ve
CMV IgM	−ve	+ve
Toxoplasma IgG	−ve	−ve
Toxoplasma IgM	−ve	−ve

On booking bloods, IgG was positive for rubella, HSV and VZV indicating previous exposure. The negative rubella, HSV and VZV IgM suggest exposure was not recent. For rubella and VZV, this implies immunity. HSV IgG does not necessarily provide immunity, as it does not distinguish between HSV-1 and 2. Similarly there is still the risk of reactivation of latent HSV. When compared to bloods taken at this visit, there is evidence of seroconversion for CMV IgG, suggesting primary infection has occurred between these two samples. The IgM is positive, supporting recent infection.

CMV is a ubiquitous herpes virus that usually causes a mild or asymptomatic infection in the immune competent. Occasionally primary infection causes a syndrome of infectious mononucleosis, similar to that caused by Epstein-Barr virus (EBV), with features such as sore throat, fever, fatigue, petechial rash, hepatitis, splenomegaly, haemolysis and atypical lymphocytes. It is commonly acquired through sharing saliva, although it is also spread through blood, semen, breast milk and vaginal fluid. It is an infection of childhood, particularly in less-developed countries, where over 90% are infected in childhood compared to around 40% in developed countries. Like all herpes viruses, infection can reactivate, although this tends to only occur in immune-compromised states.

In primary CMV infection during pregnancy, the risk of fetal infection is about 33%. Intrauterine CMV infection occurs mainly as a result of placental infection following maternal viraemia. If infected, there is a 20–25% chance of developing sequelae, 10–15% observable at birth, with 5–10% presenting later in infancy. While congenital CMV can occur at any stage of pregnancy, risk of sequelae is highest if infection occurs in the first trimester.

Confirming infection in the fetus is best made with amniocentesis looking for CMV DNA in the amniotic fluid, confirming the fetus is excreting virus. The amniotic CMV DNA viral load is important in picking up those who would otherwise be asymptomatic at birth. Certain features on fetal ultrasound may be suggestive, but are not definitively diagnostic, the most classic being periventricular cerebral calcifications.

If symptomatic at birth, the mortality rate is about 5%. Post-natal diagnosis in symptomatic babies would show some of the following signs:

- Growth restriction
- Haematological sequelae
- Thrombocytopenia and purpura
- Hepatosplenomegaly
- Lymphadenopathy
- Neurological sequelae
- Poor tone
- Seizures
- Microcephaly
- Chorioretinitis
- Cerebral calcification (classically periventricular)
- Deafness (can be a late manifestation and is the most common cause of sensorineural hearing loss)
- Pneumonitis
- Colitis
- Hepatitis

Sequelae in those presenting later in childhood are typically hearing defects or impaired intellectual performance.

Although most pregnant women with primary CMV will deliver an unaffected fetus, the option of termination should always be discussed. Routine use of antivirals in immune-competent people is rarely indicated, and none have been shown to reduce perinatal transmission. Data on use of antivirals in the treatment of intrauterine infection is lacking. Studies are underway to investigate the use of hyperimmune globulin, which aims to reduce transmission from mother to baby.

At delivery this neonate was noted to be small with microcephaly. He was jaundiced and had a papular rash and enlarged liver and spleen. Cranial ultrasound showed the intracerebral calcifications and large ventricles. Blood, urine and cerebrospinal fluid (CSF) were taken for routine testing. He had thrombocytopaenia and raised liver enzymes. CMV IgG and IgM were both positive. In neonates a positive IgG often represents maternal antibodies that have transferred transplacentally. IgM, however, is too large to pass through the placenta, so it usually represents active or recent infection. Urine, blood, and CSF CMV DNA polymerase chain reaction (PCR) were all positive.

In neonates, antiviral treatment with ganciclovir is controversial, as it can suppress the bone marrow. It is indicated only in symptomatic congenital CMV, where it cannot cure the infection, but can improve outcomes, such as lessening severity of hearing loss and improving brain growth.

KEY POINTS

- Congenital infections are infections acquired in utero or during delivery.
- CMV is a ubiquitous herpes virus that usually causes a mild or asymptomatic infection in the immune competent.
- In primary CMV infection during pregnancy, the risk of fetal infection is about 33%. If infected, there is a 20–25% chance of developing sequelae.
- After observing abnormalities on a scan, prenatal diagnosis is best made with amniocentesis looking for CMV DNA in the amniotic fluid. Post-natal diagnosis is best made looking for CMV DNA in urine, blood, and CSF.
- Routine use of antivirals in immune-competent people is rarely indicated, and none have been shown to reduce perinatal transmission.

CASE 96: A CHRONIC COUGH

A 28-year-old post-graduate student who recently arrived in the United Kingdom presents to his GP complaining of a cough productive with yellow sputum. He does not complain of haemoptysis or shortness of breath. When questioned, he also mentions some night sweats and loss of weight over the past 2 months. His symptoms failed to improve despite taking two previous courses of antibiotics prescribed by his doctor in India. He smokes 40 cigarettes a day and drinks moderate amounts of alcohol. He has no other past medical history. He denies having any contacts with the same symptoms.

Examination

Temperature 37.9°C, pulse 102 beats/min, blood pressure 110/60 mmHg. He is noted to have a previous bacillus Calmette-Guérin (BCG) scar on his left arm. Examination of the neck shows bilateral supraclavicular lymphadenopathy. Ear, nose, and throat examination is normal. Chest auscultation reveals bronchial breathing and an expiratory wheeze in the right upper lobe. He had a slightly tender liver but no evidence of jaundice or other signs of liver disease.

 INVESTIGATIONS

Radiology
He was sent for a chest x-ray, which shows right upper lobe consolidation, possibly some left upper lobe changes and a full hilar region suggesting enlarged lymph nodes.

Microbiology
Sputum was sent to the microbiology lab for further investigations. Blood cultures showed no growth. Urine pneumococcal antigen was negative.

? **QUESTIONS**

1. What is your immediate differential diagnosis?
2. How would you investigate this patient?
3. What is the pathogenesis of this disease?
4. How would you manage this patient?

ANSWERS

The differential diagnosis includes:

- *Pulmonary tuberculosis (PTB)*—Common presenting trio of chronic cough, night sweats and weight loss
- *Lymphoma*—Lymphadenopathy, weight loss and night sweats
- *Bronchiectasis/chronic obstructive pulmonary disease (COPD)*—Secondary to his smoking history
- *Lung cancer*—The patient is young for this diagnosis, but his smoking history would fit signs and symptoms
- Recurrent right upper lobe pneumonia

Patients who are suspected of having active PTB must have a posterior-anterior chest radiograph. This is to reveal typical changes found in TB, which classically include enlarged hilar and mediastinal lymph nodes and mid-lobe or upper lobe consolidation or cavitation.

At least three sputum samples should be sent for acid-fast bacilli (AFB) TB microscopy and culture. In a positive microscopy test (Figure 96.1) the TB bacillus displays a red stain resulting from its wall retaining the acid of the stain, thus called 'acid-fast'. If it is not possible to obtain spontaneously produced sputum, the patient should be referred for a bronchoscopy, where the lungs are washed out in an attempt to find the bacillus. If respiratory samples come back negative but you still have a high index of suspicion, immune-based tests could be performed. These include the Mantoux test or the more recent interferon gamma release assay (IGRA) tests and are a sign of previous exposure to TB. They are relatively non-specific and do not distinguish between active and past infection.

The gold standard for diagnosis is culturing the causative organism. This takes a long time, as the organism is slow growing. Historically this took up to 40 days of culture in specialised media, but newer systems have reduced this time, and culture may be positive within 2 weeks. Culture positivity is important in order to obtain antibiotic susceptibilities of the TB isolate. Molecular testing (polymerase chain reaction [PCR]) can be performed looking for TB DNA in the sample; however, sensitivity is not high enough to rule out the diagnosis if a test is negative. Molecular testing does not provide full susceptibility results, which are important for treatment.

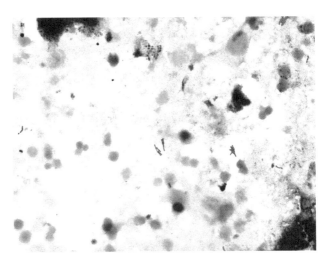

Figure 96.1 Acid-fast bacilli (red) in sputum sample.

TB can cause a disseminated illness and is not necessarily confined to the respiratory tract. Other presentations of TB include lymphadenitis, meningitis, bone and joint infections and gastrointestinal and genitourinary tract infections. Microbiological samples should be taken from appropriate sites.

TB is spread from person to person through the air. When a person with infectious pulmonary TB coughs or sneezes, tiny particles containing *Mycobacterium tuberculosis* are expelled. These particles, called droplet nuclei, are about 1–5 microns in diameter and can remain suspended in the air for several hours. If another person inhales air that contains these droplet nuclei, they reach the alveoli, and transmission of infection may occur. Not everyone who is exposed to an infectious TB patient becomes infected. The risk depends on how infectious the patient is, the duration of exposure, the virulence of the TB strain and the immune status of the contact person.

In the alveoli, some of the tubercle bacilli are killed, but a few multiply and disseminate. Bacilli may reach any part of the body, including areas where disease is likely to develop, such as upper portions of the lungs, kidneys, brain and bone. The spread and multiplication are stopped within 2–8 weeks by the body's immune response. At this time, the person has what is known as latent TB infection (LTBI). LTBI means that bacilli are in the body but the immune system is keeping them under control and inactive.

Some people with LTBI develop TB disease. TB disease develops when the immune system cannot keep the bacilli under control and they begin to multiply rapidly. The risk of developing TB disease is highest in the first 2 years after infection.

If active PTB is suspected and the patient is very unwell, treatment should be commenced without waiting for the culture results. Once a diagnosis is made, the patient should be transferred to the care of a physician with experience managing pulmonary TB. If hospital admission is needed, patients should be admitted to a single isolation room under respiratory precautions, and if suspicion of drug-resistant TB exists, they should be admitted to a negative-pressure side room. This is to reduce the spread of infection to others. All patients with TB should have an HIV test performed. All close contacts should be screened to see if transmission has occurred.

The standard treatment regimen comprises quadruple therapy with rifampicin, isoniazid, ethambutol and pyrazinamide. Pyrazinamide and ethambutol are stopped after 2 months and rifampicin and isoniazid continued for a further 4 months, to complete 6 months in total of treatment for PTB. Treatment with multiple drugs is used to reduce the development of resistance in the TB bacillus during treatment. TB should never be treated with only one antibiotic.

🔑 KEY POINTS

- PTB commonly presents as the trio of chronic cough, night sweats and weight loss.
- Diagnosis is based on clinical suspicion, typical changes on a chest x-ray and a positive AFB microscopy on respiratory (or other clinical) samples. The gold standard for diagnosis is culturing the causative organism.
- TB is spread from person to person through the air by TB-containing particles, called droplet nuclei. Not everyone who is exposed to an infectious TB patient becomes infected.
- If hospital admission is needed, patients should be admitted to a single isolation room under respiratory precautions.
- Standard treatment is quadruple therapy initially. Treatment with multiple drugs is used to reduce the development of resistance in the TB bacillus during treatment.

CASE 97: A JAUNDICED VIEW

A 31-year-old known intravenous drug user (IVDU) is admitted to hospital after a presumed drug overdose. There is no history available from the patient, and she has no medical records at this hospital.

Examination

Her Glasgow Coma Scale (GCS) is 12, but there is no meningism or localising signs. She is haemodynamically stable with a blood pressure of 105/70 mmHg. She has poor oral hygiene and is missing most of her teeth. She has a number of tattoos, some of which looked self-made. Her arms are covered in needle track marks. There is no evidence of trauma.

Her abdomen is soft and mildly tender in the right upper quadrant. The rest of the examination is within normal limits.

INVESTIGATIONS

Bloods

		Reference values
Haemoglobin	10.8 g/dL	11.4–15.0 g/dL
White cell count	13.5 × 10⁹/L	3.9–10.6 g/dL
Platelets	408 × 10⁹/L	150–440 × 10⁹/L
Urea	2.1 mmol/L	2.5–7.8 mmol/L
Creatinine	98 µmol/L	45–90 µmol/l
Bilirubin	46 µmol/L	<21 µmol/L
ALT	270 IU/L	<40 IU/L
AST	170 IU/L	5–40 IU/L
ALP	80 IU/L	40–129 IU/L
C-reactive protein	25 mg/L	<5 mg/L

Virology

HIV	Negative
Hepatitis B sAg (HBsAg)	Positive
Hepatitis B sAb (anti-HBs)	Negative
Hepatitis B core IgM (anti-IgM)	Negative
Hepatitis B core total Ab (anti-HBc)	Positive
Hepatitis B eAg (HBeAg)	Negative
Hepatitis B eAb (anti-HBe)	Positive
Hepatitis C IgG	Negative

Radiology
CT brain showed no abnormalities.

? QUESTIONS

1. How would you interpret the results?
2. How would you manage this patient?
3. How could this infection have been prevented?

DOI: 10.1201/9781003242697-101

ANSWERS

Patients with a history of IVDU are at risk of acquiring blood-borne viruses and should be investigated for HIV and viral hepatitis.

This patient's results show mildly elevated ALT, AST, and bilirubin and a normal ALP. This suggests hepatocyte damage rather than an obstructive jaundice. The enzymes are only mildly raised, suggesting a chronic rather than acute hepatic process.

Viral serology testing excludes HIV and hepatitis C infection but confirms the presence of hepatitis B infection. Hepatitis B infection is spread parenterally, sexually and vertically. It has an incubation period of approximately 3 months, after which the symptoms of acute hepatitis occur. In the majority of cases this is cleared by the immune system. In 5–10% of infected persons, failure to clear the virus occurs and a chronic infectious state ensues. Hepatitis B infection is also causally associated with hepatocellular carcinoma. Hepatitis C virus is a widely spread RNA virus with similar transmission routes to hepatitis B, although mainly spread parenterally through blood in transfusions (before screening) and needle sharing (tattoos, IVDU). Patients with hepatitis C are more prone to developing a chronic infection and cirrhosis than those infected with other forms of hepatitis.

Serological markers are the mainstay of diagnosis of viral hepatitis (Figures 97.1 and 97.2). After acute infection, the first marker to appear in the blood is hepatitis B surface antigen (HBsAg), and looking for this antigen is the initial test done when screening for hepatitis B infection. It is part of the surface protein and reflects the presence of the virus in the blood. It is positive in acute and chronic infection and only becomes negative if the infection is cleared. If it is positive for longer than 6 months, the infection is classed as a chronic infection.

Anti-HBs, an antibody to this surface antigen, is produced as the HBsAg wanes. It represents late acute infection or past infection and the clearance of surface antigen. Positive anti-HBs can also represent vaccination, as hepatitis B vaccine contains recombinant HBsAg. In chronic infection, when HBsAg remains positive, anti-HBs will not be produced.

The nucleocapsid of the virus is reflected in two antigens, HBcAg and HBeAg.

Core antigen (HBcAg) is not measurable, as it remains inside the virus, but both IgM (anti-IgM) and IgG (anti-HBc) antibodies to HBcAg are produced and can be measured. As with other infections, IgM is produced during acute infection and will also remain positive in chronic active hepatitis, as the virus is still present. It will disappear once core antigen is no longer present, that is, once the virus has been cleared. IgG, on the other hand (as with other infections), will be produced throughout infection and remain positive after recovery as a marker of previous infection. IgG antibodies therefore do not distinguish between recent, chronic, or previous infection. If negative, however, they exclude hepatitis B infection.

HBeAg, which is a soluble part of the core antigen, can leave the virus and can therefore be measured. Its presence reflects actively replicating virus, and it will disappear when the virus stops replicating. A positive result therefore indicates acute infection or chronic active infection, implying actively replicating virus and thus high infectivity. Analogous to anti-HBs and HBsAg, anti-HBe is produced as HBeAg wanes and reflects the ceasing of active viral replication. A positive result for anti-HBe represents previous infection, or chronic, non-active hepatitis B.

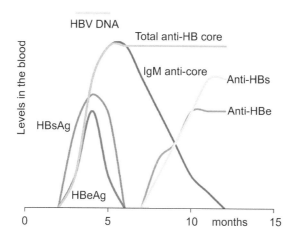

Figure 97.1 Hepatitis B viral antigens and antibodies detectable in the blood following acute infection and resolution.

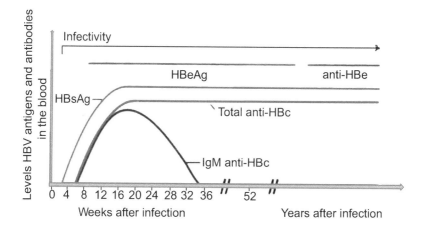

Figure 97.2 Hepatitis B viral antigens and antibodies detectable in the blood following acute infection which becomes chronic.

This patient's results therefore suggest a chronic, non-active hepatitis B infection, also known as a carrier state. A viral polymerase chain reaction (PCR) for hepatitis B virus (HBV) DNA should be done in all chronic infections to evaluate for viral replication. A liver biopsy should be considered in chronic hepatitis with a positive HBV DNA.

The other hepatitis viruses include hepatitis A–E and G (GB-V). Despite their structural differences and modes of transmission, they all target the liver cells. The vowels (A and E) are transmitted via the faecal-oral route, are usually associated with travel, and cause an acute infection presenting as gastroenteritis and hepatitis. They do not cause any chronic disease.

Most patients with hepatitis B will resolve their infection without any specific treatment. Patients in whom treatment is recommended include those who have evidence of viral replication. Treatment options currently include interferon and antiviral agents. Patient education is very important, as prevention of transmission to other people can be achieved only by collaboration with the patient.

Prevention of infection is best achieved through vaccination, which is recommended for all at risk, such as health care workers, emergency service workers, IVDUs, household members of carriers, post-exposure prophylaxis if non-immune, travellers to high-risk areas and those on renal dialysis. The vaccine contains the HBsAg and is prepared by recombinant DNA technology. It is usually given in three doses over a period of 6 months; however, this can be expedited to 2 months for patients at high risk of infection. It is important to test for seroconversion after vaccination, as some people do not produce antibodies and are therefore not protected.

🔑 KEY POINTS

- Intravenous drug users are at risk of acquiring blood-borne viruses and should be investigated for HIV and viral hepatitis.
- Hepatitis B is spread parenterally, sexually and vertically. It has an incubation period of approximately 3 months, after which the symptoms occur.
- HBsAg is the first marker to appear after acute infection and the first test done when screening for hepatitis B. Anti-HBs appears in late acute infection and remains positive. It can also represent immunity from vaccination as the hepatitis B vaccine contains recombinant HBsAg.
- Most patients with hepatitis B will resolve their infection without any specific treatment. In 5–10% of infected persons, failure of clearance of the virus occurs and a chronic state ensues. It is also causally associated with hepatocellular carcinoma.
- Prevention of infection is best achieved through vaccination, which is recommended for all at risk.

CASE 98: GRAM-NEGATIVE BACTERAEMIA

A 29-year-old man presents to the emergency department complaining of fever, headache, and malaise over the past couple of days. His symptoms are associated with nausea and abdominal pain but no diarrhoea. He has no dysuria, haematuria, or frequency and has not noticed any rash. He returned 4 days ago from a trip to Bangladesh, where he was visiting family. He noticed some mosquito bites and ate at a lot of fast-food restaurants during his stay. He has no other significant medical history and is usually fit and well.

Examination

His temperature is 39.5°C, blood pressure 130/80 mmHg and heart rate 70 beats/min. There is no rash. He has inflamed tonsils, but no spots or rash on the mucous membranes. His chest is clear. His abdomen is slightly tender, but no masses or organomegaly is found.

It was felt that he was not very unwell, and so he was discharged from the emergency department on oral co-amoxiclav after bloods were taken.

INVESTIGATIONS

Bloods		Reference values
Haemoglobin	14.8 g/dL	11.4–15.0 g/dL
White cell count	5.1×10^9/L	3.9–10.6 g/dL
Platelets	102×10^9/L	150–440 $\times 10^9$/L
Urea	5.3 mmol/L	2.5–7.8 mmol/L
Creatinine	89 µmol/L	45–90 µmol/l
Bilirubin	27 µmol/L	<21 µmol/L
ALT	67 IU/L	<40 IU/L
ALP	69 IU/L	40–129 IU/L
C-reactive protein	100 mg/L	<5 mg/L
Blood film	No malaria parasites seen	
ICT for malaria (antigen test)	Negative	

Microbiology

1. Blood cultures after 24 hours flagged up positive. Gram stain showed Gram-negative rods.
2. Urine MC&S: Negative.

QUESTIONS

1. What is your differential diagnosis based on the above findings?
2. What would be your management plan?
3. What is the pathogenesis of this infection?
4. What further tests and investigations would you request on this patient?

ANSWERS

In a returning traveller from Bangladesh presenting with a fever, malaria, typhoid fever, other food-borne pathogens, dengue, arboviruses and hepatitis should be considered. HIV should also be considered if risk is established. It is important to remember non-travel-related common infections, such as urinary tract infection, inflammatory bowel disease and cholecystitis, that might present similarly.

The blood culture result narrows the diagnosis to conditions caused by a Gram-negative bacteraemia. From this, typhoid and paratyphoid are most likely, but it could still be a common pathogen such as *Escherichia coli* secondary to a non-travel-related cause.

Enteric fever (sometimes known as typhoid fever) is caused by the Gram-negative pathogens *Salmonella enterica* serotypes Typhi and Paratyphi. Transmission of the infection is via the faecal-oral route, and the disease is more common in areas where water, food and hand hygiene are poor. Humans are the only known reservoir for *S. enterica* Typhi and *S. enterica* Paratyphi.

It presents in young adults with a high-grade fever, abdominal pain, and a relative bradycardia, as is seen in this patient. One would expect a faster heart rate with such a high temperature; however, this is not the case in this patient. In addition, patients usually present with a relatively low or a normal white cell and platelet count. Impaired liver function tests are also a common finding.

While uncommon, severe complications can occur. These include intestinal haemorrhage from congested Peyer's patches, intestinal perforation, encephalitis, neuropsychiatric symptoms and metastatic abscesses.

Patients who are suspected of having typhoid fever should be started on antibiotics, which can be oral or intravenous depending on their clinical condition. Prior to commencing therapy, however, blood and stool cultures should be sent to the microbiology laboratory. Initial choice of therapy depends on the susceptibility patterns of the pathogen in the area it was acquired, as some geographic regions have high resistance to certain antibiotics. Intravenous ceftriaxone is currently the treatment of choice. Oral options for treatment include ciprofloxacin and azithromycin, but should be prescribed only once testing has confirmed they are sensitive. The duration of treatment varies from 7 to 14 days.

The fever usually resolves within 4 days of appropriate therapy, but may last longer. Prolonged fever is not necessarily a sign of complicated disease.

As salmonellae are highly infectious, all patients should be admitted to an isolation room and enteric precautions undertaken to prevent spread of the infection to other patients. Health authorities responsible for public health and epidemiology, such as the Public Health England, should be notified.

Following ingestion, the organism reaches the intestinal mucosa, where it attaches to the M cells of the Peyer's patches, which have a wide array of molecules that assist in the attachment and invasion of the intestinal barrier. The organism causes systemic infection by crossing the gastrointestinal epithelial barrier to invade the macrophages at the submucosal space. Despite the hostile environment within the macrophage, they are able to survive and replicate. The inflammatory response mounted by the host is partially due to activation of the innate immune response.

A small number of people, called carriers, recover from typhoid fever but continue to carry the bacteria. Both ill persons and carriers shed *Salmonella* Typhi in their faeces (stool). Stool should be tested to ensure clearance of carriage, especially in those working as food handlers or with vulnerable groups of people.

This patient could have benefited from vaccination prior to travel. Two types of vaccines are currently available for typhoid: a live oral attenuated vaccine and a parenteral polysaccharide vaccine. They protect only against *S.* Typhi and not against *S.* Paratyphi, so food hygiene precautions also should be recommended to all travellers to endemic areas.

> 🔑 **KEY POINTS**
>
> - Typhoid fever (also known as enteric fever) is caused by the Gram-negative pathogens *S. enterica* serotypes Typhi and Paratyphi. Transmission of the infection is via the faecal-oral route.
> - Typhoid fever usually presents in young adults with a high-grade fever and non-specific symptoms.
> - Initial choice of therapy depends on the susceptibility patterns of the pathogen in the area it was acquired. Intravenous ceftriaxone is currently the treatment of choice.
> - Both ill persons and carriers shed *Salmonella* Typhi in their faeces. Thus testing is important in those working as food handlers or health care professionals.

CASE 99: A GROIN SWELLING

A 42-year-old intravenous drug user (IVDU) is admitted to hospital complaining of fever and a painful left groin. She has been injecting for a number of years and has had multiple hospital admissions for infected injection sites. She is currently injecting into the left groin. She denies any other symptoms.

Examination

She is underweight and has poor personal hygiene. She has a fever (temperature 39.2°C), her pulse is 130 beats/min, and blood pressure is 100/70 mmHg. Respiratory and cardiovascular examinations are unremarkable, and her abdomen is soft and non-tender. Her arms are scarred from previous injections, and her skin shows evidence of excoriations from chronic scratching. A left inguinal swelling is noted, being hot, red and painful to the touch. There is cellulitis surrounding the swollen area.

Routine bloods and blood cultures are taken, and she is started empirically on IV benzylpenicillin and flucloxacillin for her abscess and cellulitis. Surgery is planned to drain the abscess.

🔍 INVESTIGATIONS

Bloods

		Reference values
Haemoglobin	11.0 g/dL	11.4–15.0 g/dL
White cell count	20.0×10^9/L	3.9–10.6 g/dL
Platelets	340×10^9/L	$150–440 \times 10_9$/L
C-reactive protein	184 mg/L	<5 mg/L

Microbiology

MRSA screen: Negative.
Pus from the abscess grew methicillin-resistant *Staphylococcus aureus* (MRSA) and *Streptococcus pyogenes* (group A streptococcus).

? QUESTIONS

1. What is the most likely diagnosis?
2. Is her current antibiotic treatment adequate?
3. What infection control measures are required in hospital?
4. What is the pathogenesis of the toxic shock syndrome caused by both *Staphylococcus aureus* and *Streptococcus pyogenes*?

ANSWERS

An abscess is a localised collection of pus (neutrophils) that is a result of the inflammatory response to a bacterial infection or a foreign body. Certain bacteria are more likely to result in abscesses, such as staphylococci. The immune system reaction to the bacteria is protective and tries to prevent the infection from spreading. This results in a collection of bacteria, inflammatory cells, and debris. This presents as an area of fluctuance and pain, usually with surrounding cellulitis and overlying skin erythema and heat. There may also be associated systemic signs such as fever, raised inflammatory markers and bacteraemia. The most common causes of skin and soft tissue infection are *S. aureus* and *S. pyogenes*.

Both *S. aureus* and *S. pyogenes* cause invasive disease and significant morbidity and mortality. Invasive disease may take the form of severe spreading skin and soft tissue infection (including necrotising fasciitis), disseminated infection and toxic shock syndrome.

Imaging of the groin should be performed to exclude deep-seated infection that may be present, such as a pelvic or thigh abscess or osteomyelitis. Imaging of the surrounding tissue is needed to exclude necrotising fasciitis if the pain is severe or cellulitis continues to spread despite adequate treatment.

S. aureus is associated with pus- and abscess-forming infection of skin and soft tissues, especially if medical devices such as cannulae or catheters are present. It is also the cause of significant infections of bone and joints, heart and other organs to which it disseminates. A more serious form of infection, such as necrotising pneumonia, necrotising fasciitis, and severe sepsis, occurs in strains possessing the genes for Panton-Valentine leukocidin (PVL) toxin. Aside from the presence of medical devices, invasive disease does not require risk factors and occurs in young, otherwise healthy individuals.

S. pyogenes (group A streptococcus [GAS]) is most commonly associated with 'strep throat' and skin and soft tissue infection such as impetigo, erysipelas and cellulitis. Less common complications include necrotising fasciitis, scarlet fever, rheumatic fever and post-streptococcal glomerulonephritis. Invasive disease occurs most commonly in people with risk factors, such as extreme age, recent childbirth, IVDU, alcoholism, diabetes, cancer and immune suppression.

Abscesses are best treated by incision and drainage to remove the source of infection.

Penicillin or flucloxacillin is appropriate treatment for GAS, but MRSA will not be adequately treated. If GAS infection is severe, the antibiotic clindamycin should be added. Aside from killing the bacterium directly, it has an added effect of reducing toxin production, therefore reducing much of the toxin-mediated tissue damage associated with severe disease.

MRSA is an *S. aureus* strain that is resistant to the ß-lactam group of antibiotics, which include penicillins, cephalosporins, and carbapenems. It is often resistant to other groups of antibiotics such as the aminoglycosides, macrolides, and quinolones, making it more difficult to treat. It causes the same infections as methicillin-sensitive *S. aureus* (MSSA). Treatment for MRSA has a limited range of antibiotics, including the glycopeptides (e.g., vancomycin), linezolid, daptomycin, tetracyclines, fusidic acid and rifampicin, often used in combination to reduce the risk of further resistance developing. The patient's antibiotic treatment should thus be changed to include one of these, some of which will also treat the GAS. An example of a treatment regimen would be vancomycin plus clindamycin.

MRSA colonisation and infection are also treated with a decolonisation regimen to attempt to reduce the burden of MRSA present and to reduce the risk of developing further infection. This regimen includes an antiseptic body wash and nasal application of an antibiotic or antiseptic.

Both MRSA and GAS can spread between patients and from patients to staff, causing outbreaks. To prevent this, this patient should be admitted into a single room for isolation. Precautions to reduce the risk of spread include the use of personal protective equipment (PPE) for any health care worker having contact with her or her immediate environment. The PPE includes the use of gloves and aprons and face protection if aerosols are to be generated, such as for wound dressings and suctioning. Hand washing with soap and water or decontaminating hands with an alcohol-based hand rub is recommended before and after contact with her or her immediate environment.

Among the many virulence factors of cell surface antigens, capsule, adhesins, and toxins, are the group known as streptococcal pyrogenic exotoxins (SPE), previously called erythrogenic toxins. These SPE (A, B, and C) act as superantigens, in that they are able to directly and non-specifically stimulate T cells of the immune system, resulting in massive cytokine production, leading to fever, muscle lysis, severe sepsis, and shock. In *S. aureus* the same process occurs in response to the exotoxin toxic shock syndrome toxin-1 (TSST-1).

🔑 KEY POINTS

- Abscesses are localised collections of pus (neutrophils) developing in response to bacterial infection.
- The most common causes of skin and soft tissue infection are *S. aureus* and *S. pyogenes*. *S. aureus* is associated with pus- and abscess-forming infection of skin and soft tissues, especially if medical devices such as cannulae or catheters are present.
- Abscesses are best treated by incision and drainage to remove the source of infection.
- MRSA is *S. aureus* that is resistant to the ß-lactam group of antibiotics, which includes penicillins, cephalosporins and carbapenems.

A 24-year-old man is referred to the local genitourinary medicine (GUM) clinic. He has been complaining of recent onset of dysuria and has also noticed a yellowish urethral discharge. He denies any constitutional symptoms, frequency, or haematuria. He has not noticed any rash, conjunctivitis or joint pains. His background history is unremarkable. He is heterosexual with a number of sexual partners and practices unsafe sex.

Examination

General examination is normal. There is a small amount of muco-purulent discharge evident from the urethra, which was mildly erythematous around the meatus.

There is no rash visible, nor any evidence of genital ulceration or inguinal lymphadenopathy. The testes and prostate are non-tender and not enlarged.

Urine and urethral swabs are taken for investigation. Due to his risky sexual behaviour, blood is taken for syphilis, HIV, and hepatitis B. A list of his sexual contacts is requested for contact tracing.

🔍 INVESTIGATIONS

Microbiology
Urethral swab

	Microscopy (performed in the clinic)	WBC +++
		Epithelial cells ++ Intracellular diplococci (coffee bean shaped)
	Microscopy (performed in the lab)	WBC +++
		Epithelial cells ++ Gram-negative intracellular diplococci

Culture: *Neisseria gonorrhoeae*
Urine MC&S

	Microscopy	WBC +++ RBC + Epithelial cells + Bacteria +++

Culture: No growth
Urine nucleic acid amplification test (NAAT): Positive for *N. gonorrhoeae*, negative for *Chlamydia trachomatis*

❓ QUESTIONS

1. What is the differential diagnosis for urethral discharge?
2. How is this condition diagnosed?
3. How would you manage this patient?

ANSWERS

The differential diagnosis of urethral discharge is classically divided into gonococcal urethritis (GU) and non-gonococcal urethritis (NGU).

GU is a sexually transmitted infection caused by the Gram-negative diplococcus *Neisseria gonorrhoeae*. There is generally a short history of dysuria and a thick urethral discharge occurring after a recent contact. In women, the presentation can be slower and may be asymptomatic. Disseminated infection occurs if the organism spreads to the systemic circulation. This is characterised by fever, rash and suppurative arthritis.

NGU presentation tends to be more indolent, with a 3- to 4-week history being usual. The dysuria and discharge are less prominent, and the discharge is waterier than for GU. Causes of NGU include:

- *Chlamydia trachomatis*, the most common cause of sexually transmitted infection reported in the UK, especially in young adults and adolescents. Symptoms may come and go over several weeks, and it may appear to spontaneously resolve in some. It may also be asymptomatic, especially in women. There is co-infection with *N. gonorrhoeae* in about 20% of patients, and empiric treatment will usually treat both these infections simultaneously.
- *Mycoplasma genitalium*, emerging as a common cause of NGU, and is more commonly symptomatic than *C. trachomatis*. It is more difficult to diagnose and is therefore sometimes treated empirically.
- *Trichomonas vaginalis* infection, a common cause of vaginitis in women and also an important source of urethritis in men. A 22% urethral prevalence was found among male partners of women with known trichomonal infection. The condition should be suspected in patients with symptoms but little or no discharge on physical examination.
- *Ureaplasma urealyticum*, more recently thought to be a cause of NGU. It may account for 10–40% of NGU cases and is sexually transmitted.
- Herpes simplex virus infection, most often associated with painful superficial genital ulcers that are usually visible on the external genitalia.
- Prostatitis, especially in older men with enlarged prostates, predisposing to obstruction and infection. Minor penile discharge may be present. Symptoms of urinary outflow obstruction and perineal discomfort may be the predominant symptoms.

No test is currently 100% sensitive or specific for *N. gonorrhoeae*. Routine urine microscopy, culture, and sensitivity (MC&S) culture media does not support its growth. Options for diagnosis of urethritis are microscopy, culture and molecular tests:

- *Microscopy*: Staining of the urethral discharge is helpful in looking for pus cells, as well as the typical intracellular, bean-shaped diplococci of *N. gonorrhoeae*. If a Gram stain is performed, the bacteria will look pink in colour (Gram negative). Microscopy has a sensitivity of 90–95% in symptomatic men for *N. gonorrhoeae*. Sensitivity is poor for endocervical (<50%), rectal, and throat swabs and in asymptomatic men (50–75%).
- *Culture*: Using specific selective media, *N. gonorrhoeae* will grow if plated soon after the specimen is taken. It is a fragile organism, and a delay in the specimen reaching the lab will result in a false-negative culture, as it will have died en route. Thus some GUM clinics plate the specimens directly onto culture plates in the clinic. It is not practical to culture for *Chlamydia* or *Ureaplasma* because it is technically difficult, takes 2–3 days to get a result, and is expensive.

- *Molecular tests*: Nucleic acid amplification test (NAAT) is the standard diagnostic and screening test used for *N. gonorrhoeae* and *C. trachomatis*. It is >96% sensitive even on asymptomatic cases and can be performed on swabs from any site as well as urine samples from men. Sensitivity on urine samples from women is significantly lower than from an endocervical swab and is not recommended.

N. gonorrhoeae has become significantly resistant to a spectrum of antibiotics. There are no longer any oral antibiotics that can be recommended alone for first-line treatment with the certainty of curing the infection. First-line treatment for uncomplicated gonococcal infection is currently a single dose of parenteral ceftriaxone with oral azithromycin. The azithromycin is thought to have a synergistic effect with the cephalosporin, and is also used to try to delay emergence of resistance to the cephalosporin. Testing for cure and contact tracing is recommended after treatment.

KEY POINTS

- GU causes a mucopurulent urethral discharge in men and endocervical infection in women.
- NGU presentation tends to be more indolent, with less prominent dysuria and waterier discharge than GU. The most common cause of NGU is *C. trachomatis*.
- NAAT is the current standard test for symptomatic and asymptomatic *N. gonorrhoeae*.
- *N. gonorrhoeae* is becoming multi-drug resistant, with current recommendation for treatment of uncomplicated infection being parenteral cephalosporin with oral azithromycin.

INDEX

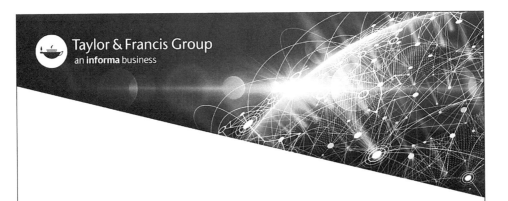
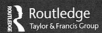
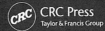